☐ PLAN

☐ PREP

☑ EAT

☐ REPEAT

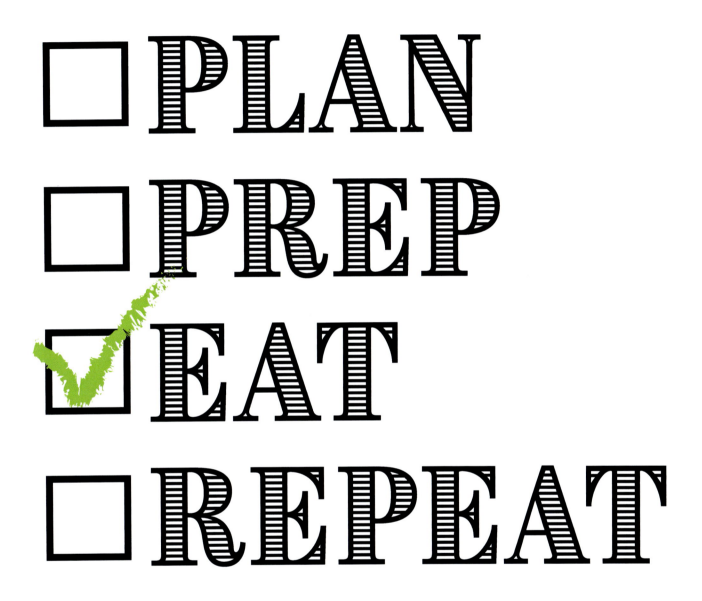

☐ PLAN
☐ PREP
☑ EAT
☐ REPEAT

Eat Better. Look Better. Feel Better.

Michelle Keyes

Copyright © 2017 Michelle Keyes

Book Design: Camilo A. Monroy

All rights reserved. This book or any portion thereof
may not be reproduced or used in any manner whatsoever
without the express written permission of the publisher
except for the use of brief quotations in a book review.

ISBN 978-1-979-79189-2

Michelle Keyes
www.thekeyesingredients.com

First Printing, 2017

Printed in the United States of America

To my devoted husband Kevin, for his endless support and encouragement, and my favorite side-kicks, my son Carson and daughter Isabella, for their creative contributions to our meals and this book.

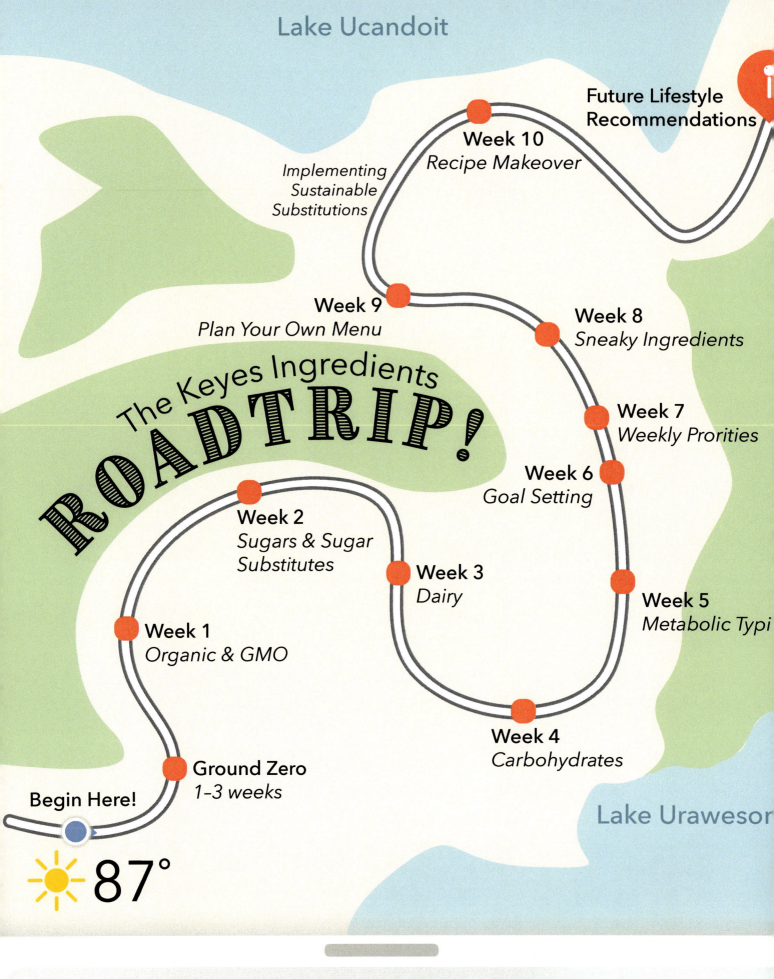

CONTENTS

1	About This Book
3	Welcome!
4	Nutrition 101
9	Let's Talk About You
13	Setting You Up for Success
16	Great Expectations
20	Phase 1 Declutter (Ground Zero)
24	Grocery Shop & Chop
27	Your Keyes to Eating Out
30	Phase 2 Detoxify (Weeks 1 & 2)
44	Phase 3 Delicious (Weeks 3 & 4)
59	Metabolically Speaking
66	Phase 4 Differentiate (Weeks 5-8)
80	Phase 5 Defy the Norm (Weeks 9, 10 & Beyond)
83	Ultimate Kitchen List
85	Meal Planner
86	Daily Journal
87	Questionnaire Key
90	References
91	Quick Tips
95	Menu

For recipes visit www.thekeyesingredients.com

ABOUT THIS BOOK

WHO CARES THIS MUCH ABOUT FOOD & WHY?

You may wonder who spends so much time researching food? Learning about my journey as a mother and educator may help you understand my passion for healthy living.

Growing up in Ontario, Canada with an Italian father and an Irish mother who learned to cook Italian meant spending a lot of time in the kitchen. Meals were made from scratch and hours were spent rolling out homemade pasta, stirring tomato sauce with love and taste-testing my grandmother's famous chocolate éclair recipe to try to find the missing mystery ingredient.

My affection for cooking was instilled at a very young age and continued into adulthood as I went off to school to pursue a degree in Psychology and Education. Along the way, I was fortunate to meet a man who shared the same appetite for food and learning as I do. I followed him and a trail of hot sauce to Texas after getting married. He set up practice as a chiropractor while I taught middle and high school and coached running.

Little did I know, I would soon be embarking upon the most important career of my life: parenting my son Carson and daughter Isabella. As with all young families, life was very busy, so I put teaching on hold to be with our children. I still made homemade meals, but often the time spent and nutrient content was less than desirable. Our diet consisted of a variety of meats, fruits, vegetables and dairy, and occasionally we went out to eat. I believed our family was healthy.

It was not until Carson started to suffer from chronic sinus congestion at the age of three that we knew something was wrong. After trying the typical drugstore variety of children's decongestants, and homeopathic remedies, we consulted an ear, nose and throat specialist. It was decided that Carson was to have his adenoids removed and tubes placed in his ears. Below is a journal entry from the day of his surgery.

Thursday, April 19th, 2007
Carson is scheduled for adenoid surgery at seven o'clock a.m. He has been having trouble smelling, hearing and breathing lately. He used to have a very keen sense of smell and always ask, "What do I smell cooking, Mommy?" I have not heard these words in what seems like forever, instead they have been replaced with "Pardon me?" due to his lack of hearing. Carson has been very clingy, especially at bedtime. He wants me to sleep with him, and I have been simply because he often gasps for air during the night. Kevin and I discussed what we thought was foolish worry as Carson was wheeled away to have the tubes put in and adenoids removed. This was the day that changed the rest of our lives!

Dr. Stark came into the waiting room and proceeded to tell us that Carson was fine. He went on to say it was not the adenoids that were causing the problem. His next words echoed for what seemed like an eternity—"It's a tumor." Kevin was hopeful. There are benign tumors…"Couldn't this be something benign?" he asked. Dr. Stark slowly shook his head and responded, "Not this one, not one that looks like this." Within twenty minutes, we had a preliminary diagnosis - lymphoma.

I could write a book about that time in my life, including making chemotherapy fun for a three-year-old and the hardship of our family being physically separated. However, I would rather write about how not to get there in the first place. Carson, through much prayer and medical assistance, survived both cancer and chemotherapy. I believe the treatment he received killed off his advanced stage three Burkett's Lymphoma; however, I do not believe that is what is keeping him healthy today.

Upon leaving the children's cancer clinic with my weak, thin, immunosuppressed son, I prayed that we would never do this again. The aftermath was worse for me. More scans, first every month, then every three, then every six and so on. The night before the scans was sleepless for all of us. We were six months out of treatment, supposedly "cancer free." Ironically, I felt no freedom. After a "routine" check and a set of scans that showed the cancer may have come back, I hit a turning point in my life. At this point I knew two things. The first was that I did it once; I had managed, through God's grace to get through cancer treatment with a child who deserved so much more of a life than what he had experienced. Second, I knew I was not capable of doing it again.

This is where my prayers changed. They went from "Lord, please help us to be cancer-free" to "Lord please help me learn and understand the truth." These prayers were answered and my eyes opened in a way I cannot explain. This newfound passion was burning a hole in my soul as I longed for the truth about food, nutrition, and the lifestyle that supported it. I became fascinated with the immune system. What builds it up? What tears it down? I passionately spent the next five years praying for and researching the truth about food. In discovering the truth I also found the freedom our family so desperately needed. No one in our home has lost a single night's sleep worrying if that cancer will come back. We know differently. We know the truth.

My studies have taught me many things. Things like this is a touchy and intimidating subject area. It can be overwhelming. It is best to read a wide range of opinions, research, and studies before forming your own opinion. I am not a doctor, nor a dietitian. Also, I am not someone who dwells on the "what ifs" of life. The only "what if" I am concerned about is "what if" you and your family knew what I have learned? Would it make a difference?

Some years ago, I sincerely thought I was providing good food for my family. Based on all my research, I have concluded that although I was sincere, I was sincerely wrong. Knowledge is power. I want the knowledge I have gained to make a powerful impact on your life I hope you enjoy the beautiful truth; *"La Bella Verita."*

WELCOME

We are so glad that you have joined us to begin your journey towards lifelong health in a sustainable way. The Keyes Ingredients exists to create an environment in our bodies to prevent and avoid illness, while achieving our fullest potential in all we do. We avoid refined and processed foods, thus limiting grains and dairy. Using whole foods makes our way of eating nutrient dense, anti-inflammatory, low glycemic, alkalizing, anti-cancer, immune-boosting and satiating. We use foods to fuel the body with body building elements. This way of eating, accompanied by positive thinking, makes the Keyes Ingredients protocol not a diet, but a sustainable way of eating for life.

Ground Zero is a time for you to prepare for the shift in your family's nutrition. We have asked you to prepare a few recipes this week that will allow you to be more successful as your journey continues. We know that life happens, and want to set you up for success to make it through those tough days. We are in this together, and we both have expectations. This is a real life journey, one without a destination. Adopting this lifestyle will keep you young, and like a fine bottle of wine you will get better with age.

Planning is an essential part of this journey. You will gain an immense awareness of what is in today's food. You will learn how to shop efficiently and effectively. The first phase (Ground Zero) is a time for you to mentally prepare for your exciting journey. We do not plan your meals during this time. We ask you to be mindful of your personal eating habits. We ask you to do your best to avoid anything out of a package.

The website, www.thekeyesingredients.com is a safe place to start to find great whole food recipes. The recipes on our site use sustainable substitutes enabling you to eat meals you are already eating and enjoying like Caesar salads and even pizza. Focus on eating whole foods and you will be on your way to fighting disease as opposed to feeding it.

Until we eat again,

Michelle L Keyes

NUTRITION 101

The age old question "So, what's for dinner?" has become somewhat of a brow-furrowing experience. Food and what to eat is a controversial subject today. With all the information available, it becomes overwhelming, confusing, and exhausting. I find it puzzling how such a simple concept like fueling the body has become distorted, manipulated and difficult to achieve.

We understand enough about automobiles that we would not put a foreign substance, like bird seed, in our gas tanks. We know that if you do not fuel an automobile properly, it does not function properly and eventually breaks down. When the price of gas goes up, we go to the pump, grumble a little, but we pay it.

Yet, when it comes to fueling our bodies, the "vehicle" that gets us around, we consistently choose things that cause us not to function properly. We choose things that "break us down." We spend significant time and money attempting to "tune our bodies up," however, when we go to the grocery store, we often compromise financially on the things that best fuel our bodies. I find this simple analogy quite profound.

What we eat has become so processed and chemical-ridden over the past few decades, that if we were given only the ingredient list, we would be hard pressed to identify the item. One of my favorite quotes from Michael Pollen is "If it grows on a plant, eat it. If it is made in a plant, don't." If it were only this easy. The truth is, everyBODY requires a proper balance of macronutrients. Each body differs in the balance and the ratios of these macronutrients. This metabolic concept is explained in more detail later in your journey.

At the end of the day it all boils down to choices. We all make mistakes, get off track on our food journey. Let's face it. Life happens. Here is the good news: You do not have to wait until next week, next month or next year to choose better. You can choose better at your next meal. This is your life, your health and you are worth it.

There are three macronutrients: Carbohydrates, Proteins and Fats.

CARBOHYDRATES

Carbohydrates are a necessary source of fuel for the body. Carbohydrates are found in fruits, vegetables, beans and grains. The key is deciphering complex and good quality carbohydrates from refined, empty carbohydrates.

PROTEINS

Proteins are an essential part of all living organisms. They are our body's building blocks. We ingest proteins through meats, eggs, dairy products, nuts, seeds, and some fruits and vegetables. Good quality protein builds a much stronger foundation than poor quality protein.

FATS

Fat is the most misunderstood and most important macronutrient for human development. Our brains are over 60% fat. Fat is the most preferred fuel for the brain. Without fat, your body cannot make hormones critical for human function. Last, but not least…this amazing macronutrient does many things but making you fat is NOT one of them!

Disease is caused by one of two things: toxicity or deficiency. Sometimes both. By correcting your deficiencies and reducing your toxicity you will be on your way to being well.

The following concepts have been briefly summarized, as there are several books written in depth about each topic separately. You do not need to be an expert in each area, you simply need to be aware of the topic and how it affects you and your family. We address a different theme every week. You do not need to know it all at once. Take it one bite at a time and digest. Making educated choices on what you use as fuel will help your body avoid blood sugar spikes and help you steer clear of blood sugar crashes.

ORGANIC

Organic simply means free from harmful chemicals. The very chemicals that are used to spray conventional crops are linked to numerous cancers and behavioral disorders in children. Conventional farming is not what is portrayed on the labels of the foods consumers purchase. The USDA organic label is trusted to ensure there are no GMO's used in the product. Organic farmers are kept to much stricter guidelines than other farms.

GENETICALLY MODIFIED FOODS

A genetically modified food is a food whose seed DNA has been altered in a lab. Why would anyone do that? If you could take the genes of a flounder and put it into the gene of a tomato so the tomato plant could withstand cold temperatures, why not? Changing a living thing's DNA is a bit like "playing God." Today, scientists are able to manipulate a plant's genes so it will not perish, even after it has been sprayed with harmful chemicals. GMO's have been linked to cancer, tumor growth, infertility and more. It is best for your health to avoid these foods completely. Companies do not have to label foods containing GMO's. Some companies have chosen to label their product as GMO free. Reading and understanding the labels on your foods is very important.

REFINED FOODS

Refined foods are highly processed and essentially void of nutrients. Refined foods are a poor source of energy, as they are not a quality fuel. Refined ingredients are things like refined flour and refined sugar. They make up the bulk of starches like breads, pastas, crackers, and other snack foods. They have an inflammatory effect on the body and promote disease.

GLUTEN FREE ALTERNATIVES

Beware of items labeled "gluten-free," as most are made of corn or soy flour which are both genetically modified. Gluten intolerance has increased. A large population of people are gluten intolerant (which does not mean allergic), and intolerances interfere with digestion and overall health. The best way to be gluten free is to choose foods that do not contain gluten in the first place.

SUGAR

It is everywhere and has more aliases than any other ingredient. Sugar is used to sweeten, add flavor to fat free foods, it causes cellular inflammation and is highly addictive. Yes, addictive. It lights up the same pleasure centers in the brain as cocaine. There are 600,000 packaged foods on the grocery store shelves, and 80 percent of them have added sugar. Refined foods break down as sugar and therefore have a negative effect on the body and the immune system. High Fructose Corn Syrup (HFCS) is just one of many aliases on grocery labels. It is a sneaky and cheap form of sweetness and is found in just about everything, from sodas and condiments, to "healthy" bread selections and salad dressings. It is made from genetically modified corn crops.

ARTIFICIAL SWEETENERS

They are artificial, man-made chemicals. Our bodies were not created to ingest, nor digest, these chemicals, especially in large amounts and as frequently as we do. They confuse our body's natural calorie counter. They promote migraines, cause nervous system damage, and are known carcinogens.

ARTIFICIAL ADDITIVES/PRESERVATIVES

These chemicals are derived from petroleum. The brighter the color, the more petroleum there is. Chemicals have no nutrient value. Instead, they cause nervous system malfunction and promote behavioral disorders. Artificial preservatives are carcinogenic and promote a very heavy toxic load for the liver.

HYDROGENATED OILS

Hydrogenated oil is oil boiled with metal, such as nickel, aluminum, or platinum. As it is processed in this manner, the oils' molecular structure changes. These oils are literally one molecule away from being plastic. The purpose of processing these oils is to elongate shelf life. These unhealthy oils cause nervous system disorders, promote heart disease, tumor growth, and birth defects.

SOY & SOY PRODUCTS

Soy products should be avoided, with the exception of a few naturally fermented ones, such as miso, natto and tamari (organic soy sauce). Nearly all soy is genetically modified. Presently, the FDA is not required to disclose this on the labels.

SUPPLEMENTATION

Eat right, exercise and take your vitamins. This has been wise advice for many years. Supplementing our diet is necessary today as our food quality and soil are not as they once were. Everyone's needs are different and we all require different supplementation. Eating cleaner will help with some deficiencies and toxicity. There are three supplements I feel everyone can benefit from, with quality being the upmost standard: a pharmaceutical-grade Omega 3, a probiotic and Vitamin D3.

OMEGA 3'S

Omega 3's are difficult to attain through diet alone. They are present in some fish, nuts, and seeds but hard to attain. It is wise to supplement. A healthy body maintains a proper balance of omega three and omega six. Too much omega six fatty acids lead to inflammation. Taking a good quality fish oil helps this balance.

PROBIOTICS

Our gut is our second brain. Healthy gut equals healthy body. Probiotics feed the good bacteria in our gut lining. There are many different strands of probiotics, and ingesting different strands is helpful in maintaining a good balance. Despite all the colorful ads, commercial dairy/yogurt is NOT a good source of probiotics. Kombucha (a fermented green tea) and other fermented foods are beneficial for your overall health and they are rich in probiotics, however supplementing with a reputable probiotic is still recommended.

VITAMIN D3

The sun lights up our world, and of course, is the best way to get our vitamin D naturally. Twenty minutes a day is all we need, yet most of us are horribly deficient in this necessary vitamin. Vitamin D is critical for optimal health. Vitamin D3 is a fat soluble vitamin, so it must be taken with fat. There are versions of this suspended in oil, which is convenient. I cannot stress enough the importance of quality on supplements.

WHAT ARE PURINES?

Purines are the building blocks of our DNA. They are called nucleotides. Purines break down in the body as uric acid. Some metabolisms have the ability to use high purine foods as fuel. Some metabolisms digest them with ease and feel energized. Other metabolisms do not metabolize high purine foods as well, resulting in excess uric acid in the body, often leaving them feeling sluggish in their digestion. Some people are best ingesting lower purine foods. An excess of uric acid in the body leads to health problems, such as gout. Examples of foods high in purines include organ meats, beef, bacon, pork, lamb, game meats, alcohol (especially beer), anchovies, sardines, herring, mackerel and scallops. Examples of foods include eggs most vegetables, fruits, chicken, and white fish.

LET'S TALK ABOUT YOU!

1. Is your Job…
    a. Sedentary
    b. Active
    c. Combination of both

2. Do you wake up tired?
    a. Always
    b. Sometimes
    c. Never

3. Do you eat breakfast?
    a. Daily
    b. Often
    c. Sometimes
    d. Never

4. How many meals a day do you eat?
    a. 2 Large
    b. 3 Moderate
    c. 5 Small

5. You have fixed mealtimes?
    a. Yes
    b. No
    c. Mostly

6. How often do you eat processed (boxed) foods?
    a. Several times a day
    b. Several times a week
    c. Once in a while
    d. Never

7. How many servings of fruit do you have in a day? _____

8. How many servings of vegetables do you have in a day? _____

9. Do you eat dairy products?

Yes   No

10. When consuming dairy, is it organic or raw?

Yes   No   Not Sure

11. Do you eat meat?
Yes   No

12. When you consume meats/eggs, are they farm raised or organic?
Yes   No

13. How many meals a week do you eat out? _____

14. Do you snack in between meals?
Yes   No

15. Typical snacks are:
    a. Fruits
    b. Vegetables
    c. Nuts
    d. Seeds
    e. Processed foods (boxed)
    f. Junk food (candy/chocolate)
    g. Juice
    h. Others

16. How many hours a week do you exercise? _____

17. When eating a meal, I am…
    a. Sitting with others
    b. Sitting alone
    c. Standing
    d. On the go
    e. In front of TV, computer or other media device

18. My consumption includes (check all that apply):
    a. Water
    b. Soda
    c. Diet soda
    d. Tea
    e. Coffee
    f. Juice
    g. Energy drinks

19. How many alcoholic drinks do you consume in a week? _____

20. Do you use artificial sweetener?

Yes				No

21. Do you ingest GMO's? (Genetically Modified Foods)

Yes				No			Not Sure

22. Do you like to cook?

Yes				No			Indifferent

23. How many people in your household to cook for? _____

24. Do you suffer from (circle all that apply)
    a. Gas
    b. Bloating
    c. Indigestion
    d. Digestive upset
    e. Skin rashes

25. Do you use tobacco in any form?

Yes				No

26. How many hours of sleep do you average each night? _____ Is it interrupted?   Yes   No

27. How do you cope with/manage stress?

_____

28. Do you feel you are aware of the amount of calories and/or macronutrients in food?

Yes				No

29. Are you familiar with chiropractic care?

Yes				No

PERSONAL GOALS

PHYSICAL GOALS

8 weeks:

6 months:

1 year:

EMOTIONAL GOALS

8 weeks:

6 months:

1 year:

SPIRITUAL GOALS

8 weeks:

6 months:

1 year:

SETTING YOU UP FOR SUCCESS

Let me begin by saying that there is no such thing as "healthy food," only "better ingredients." I believe you can do anything you believe you can do. I am not saying it will be easy but anything in life worth doing requires some good old effort and hard work. I think most will agree that time is a major factor in preparing healthy meals. Time is an issue, however, organizing your time to prioritize home cooked meals over take-out food is possible. Planning your meals ahead of time will give you a more detailed grocery list. It is more cost effective and you will have answered that question that rises to the top of your thought process every two to three hours during the day..."What are we having for dinner tonight?"

Kids can do a lot to help out. They can gather ingredients, mix things together, and be taught basic chopping at an early age. My children grew up in our kitchen and still love their time in there. Many hands make less work. The kitchen is a great place to bond with your children. Besides, where better for them to learn how to provide whole food, nutrient-dense balanced meals than at home? Keep in mind, if your child made dinner or helped make dinner, they will not only eat what they made, they will welcome accolades and want to do it again. Faith, food and family really do bring people together.

Different ages prefer different tasks; it is all about creating a healthy environment. My secret is putting some music on to get the party started! They come in to chat, next thing they are helping grab this and that, then chopping a thing or two. Eventually everyone is in there visiting, chopping and dancing of course. I do a bit of cooking on Saturdays. I call them "Sinatra Saturdays." Everyone makes a recipe or two, and we are prepped and ready for the week. I don't get everyone in the kitchen every week, but in our house, cooking is a team sport and listening to Ol' Blue Eyes Is Back is an added bonus. Feel free to create your own listening.

Parents, if you are wondering how to transition your picky little eaters, here are a few words to the wise. Picky eaters become problem eaters. Although young bodies are resilient and forgiving, the younger you start the better off you are. We have two choices when it comes to dinner: Take It or Leave It. Choice number two of course, comes with a side of going to bed hungry. At this point you will be called "mean," which means you are doing your job. There has never been a reported case of a child starving to death because they did not eat dinner one night. They will eat when they are hungry. They have to at least try what has been prepared. Studies have shown that if a child takes a few bites of a food (for example broccoli) every night for two weeks, the child will actually acquire a taste for it. Starting with vegetables on the sweeter side is always better.

5 SIMPLE CHANGES

I believe we all have the best intentions when it comes to eating better. Most do not know where to start. You can start with five simple changes. Make one change a week or one change a month. Taking this journey one step at a time is what will make you successful.

SIMPLE CHANGE #1
Change your salt. Substitute pink Himalayan salt for regular iodized table salt. Table salt is approximately 98% sodium chloride and 2% anti-caking agents. These anti-caking agents are chemicals and the culprit behind hypertension. Pink Himalayan salt comes from the Himalayan mountains and it is a pure substance. It has 84 minerals and trace minerals and has naturally occurring iodine.

SIMPLE CHANGE #2
Change your sugar. Substitute refined white sugar for naturally sweet alternatives like coconut sugar, maple syrup, raw honey and plant-based sweeteners such as fresh fruit or Stevia. Refined white sugar has an inflammatory effect on the body. It is highly addictive and causes our blood sugar to spike rapidly and then crash. The above substitutions are a healthier way to sweeten things without the consequences of inflammation and blood sugar spikes.

SIMPLE CHANGE #3
Change your flour. Refined white flour is in almost everything today. It has an inflammatory effect on the body and is highly addictive. It is commonly used in breads, pastas and most baked goods. Refined white flour is of course one of the biggest culprits for gluten. Gluten is harmful to our gut bacteria and many people today choose to go gluten free. We have to watch out for gluten-free products, as some of them are also made with inflammatory ingredients like corn or soy. In combination with refined sugar, refined white flour feeds disease. There are several flour substitutes readily available today. Examples of these are almond flour, coconut flour, and arrow root flour.

SIMPLE CHANGE #4
Change your oil. Our recipes use a lot of olive oil and coconut oil. It is wise to steer clear of hydrogenated and partially hydrogenated oils, vegetable oil and canola oil, which is the most commonly used oil today. It is from the rape seed and often genetically modified. These oils cause inflammation and lead to other health issues. Healthy fats are a necessity for cell reproduction and hormone production. We don't want to cut out our fat, but definitely want to choose wisely on the quality of the fats that we use in our diet.

SIMPLE CHANGE #5
Change the way you think. Before you change anything about what you eat, you will have to change the way you think about what you eat. If you associate junk food with pleasure you will crave junk food. If you learn about the effects that junk food has on the body and are able to associate junk food with negative effects, like the root cause of inflamation and disease, then you will not crave those foods.

KITCHEN TOOLS

Everyone needs the proper tools to get the job done efficiently, accurately and without any problems. These are a few of my favorite things:

- ☐ A set of good quality knives
- ☐ Variety set of kitchen utensils
- ☐ Small spatulas
- ☐ Vitamix or professional blender
- ☐ Juicer
- ☐ Chopper
- ☐ Kitchen Aid mixer
- ☐ Large measuring bowls
- ☐ Set of stainless bowls with lids
- ☐ Measuring cups and spoons
- ☐ Large cookie sheets
- ☐ Pre-cut parchment paper
- ☐ Cast iron (I love Staub) roasters and frypans
- ☐ Large stockpot (or 2)
- ☐ Vegetable spiralizer
- ☐ Crock pot
- ☐ Cutting boards
- ☐ Garlic chopper
- ☐ Designated counter top "garbage bowl"
- ☐ Cute aprons (because you will always get something on your outfit)
- ☐ Last but not least .... my little helpers in the kitchen

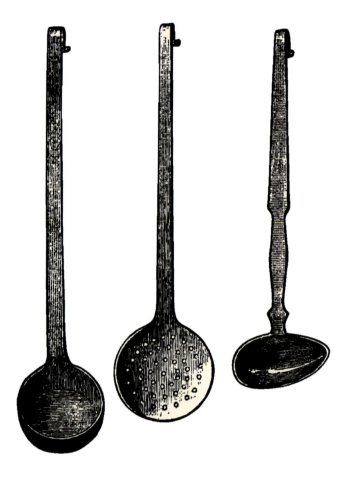

GREAT EXPECTATIONS

Embarking on something new and making a big change involves expectations. As the participant, you expect results. As the coaches, we expect you to be diligent in following our instruction. Listed below, you will find a few things you can expect in this journey.

What you can expect with our recipes:

In a nutshell, the recipes are big, bold and full of flavor. We call our recipes "Paleo Terranean." Let me explain. Basically, this means we use ingredients that have been around forever and have a Mediterranean food feel. Our menu definitely showcases quite a bit of Italian food, because well…I'm Italian and most people really do love Italian cuisine. I keep my ingredients lists short so I am not sending you out to buy everything from "A to Z" in the spice aisle. The best part is, your leftovers can be combined and go together well to make up lunch or another dinner.

Our recipes are large, or family-style, on purpose. The dinners you prepare become your lunches the next day. This is called purposeful leftovers. It works really well and is extremely efficient. Most of our soups, sauces and stews are purposefully double-batched. The intention is to eat, and then freeze it for next time. Another time saver.

Our menu is organized by week. You are given a list of meals in which you can pick and choose from, plus a grocery list and weekly prep card to help you prepare your meals in a few short hours over the weekend and have you set up for success during the week. You are also given a food list to "load up" on and one to "steer clear" of for each week. You can snap a quick picture of these lists and just keep them on their phone or tablet for convenience sake.

The first four weeks are filled with mouthwatering, EASY recipes and full of variety. Each recipe is intentionally formulated with healing ingredients. We substitute out ingredients that are harmful for viable substitutions that help heal the body. Each week will feature at least one chicken, one beef and one fish dish. We include soup and/or stew each week because they are nutrient-dense and designed to be satiating. There are plenty of options to change things up to suit your personal tastes. There are plenty of opportunities to make secondary meals out of the recipes provided. For example, using chicken carcasses/bones to make a nutrient-dense, healing broth.

The next four weeks, our menu repeats itself, with a few exceptions where we throw in some new recipes to challenge your inner chef. This, like everything else in this protocol, is done purposefully. If you are anything like me, I am always far more efficient and confident doing something for the second time, as opposed to the first. Repeating these recipes not only builds efficiency, but also builds confidence in the kitchen. The further along you get on your journey, the easier it gets! By weeks 9, 10 and beyond, you are creating your own meal plans and making substitutions based on the knowledge you have gained.

If you are cooking for three or more people, make the recipes as they are and you will have enough for your dinners and lunch the next day. If you are cooking for two people, you have options. You could divide the recipe in half, but that is never half of the work. Most couples choose menu items and repeat them, mixing it up with salads topped with a lean protein (which is always an easy fix). Some couples make the full recipe, eat half during that week, and then freeze the other half so they are prepared and have less cooking to do when the protocol repeats. If you are cooking for one, you may not have a lot of room in your freezer to freeze everything. (HINT: large ziplock freezer bags freeze and stack well.) I would encourage you to amend the family-size recipes as you see fit. I always encourage sharing and freezing extras. What a blessing you can be to a neighbor or friend by bringing them a portion of some of your healthy meals. Just don't tell them the food is healthy or they won't eat it!! Funny, but true.

Everyone is always faced with that day when things go wrong and everything unravels. This is why I highly encourage you to be prepared in advance. Freeze a small portion of stew, soup, sauce, or have an individual portion of the chicken or fish in your freezer at all times. I label these dinners "in case of emergency." At least you will have something to eat and it will deter you from going to the drive-through, which is never the window of opportunity.

What you can expect when detoxing:

Toxins are unwanted troublemakers. They are not recognized as nutrients, they hijack our hormones, and worst of all, once they enter our bodies, they are stored in our fat cells. Not cool. Detoxification means removing toxins from the body. Toxins leave the fat cells and are eliminated by sweating or using the restroom. You must stay hydrated to flush the toxins out. If the toxins are not rid from the body, they will recirculate within the body. This makes you feel, for the lack of a better word, just plain yucky! Detoxification is a process and symptoms vary for everyone.

Changes in bowel movements may occur. Constipation can be treated with our chia pudding recipe, hydrating better or by ingesting 1 tbsp of coconut oil in 4-6 oz of hot water. Frequent movements is another common symptom as we remove sugar and replace it with healthy fat. Your body will acclimate. This means that toxins are being eliminated, which is good news. If it becomes unmanageable, it can be treated by using protein shakes or chicken broth as meal replacements to give your digestive system a break.

Other detoxification symptoms include irritability, mood swings, headaches and low energy, just to name a few. In my experience, this is short-term pain for a long term gain. Detoxification juices and chicken broth help with this process.

As your journey continues, weight loss is one favorable side effect. Losing 3-4 pounds per week during detoxification is pretty typical. This would be followed by approximately one pound per week in the weeks following, until you reach your ideal weight. Here is a healthy rule of thumb. If you are trying to lose weight take your body weight and multiply by 12. The answer is the number of calories you should take in for a day. Example: if you weigh 130 pounds, multiplied by 12 would be 1,560 calories of balanced macronutrients per day. If you are maintaining a healthy weight you multiply your current body weight by 15 and that gives you the number of calories you should intake. You do not need to be weighing food nor counting every calorie. Be mindful of your general intake and the balance of your carbohydrates, proteins and fats during times you are trying to manage your body weight. You will be surprised as most people trying to lose weight often are not eating enough. This sends a final to the body to hold its fat stores.

There may come a time when the scale seems like it's frozen. There is a strategy you can use to get you over that plateau; plateaus usually happen during weeks 4 or 5. This is the time in the protocol that we evaluate your balance of macronutrients. Here is what we suggest…one day a week, you should increase your caloric and carbohydrate count. This means eating a larger portion and more carbohydrates than you have been eating, just for that day. We call this the re-feeding day.

You should not think of this as a "cheat day," because with cheating, there are always consequences. With re-feeding, therae are benefits. There is a big difference between a purposeful controlled carb intake vs. "Mc-pigging out" on harmful ingredients that will sabotage your health. The secret is to do this once a week, but no more! Use your week 4 "load up" list as your guideline.

You won't be cheating, just splurging a bit! This method is typically followed by a 1 to 2 pound weight loss in the days after.

PHASES EXPLAINED

PHASE 1: DECLUTTER

Spend a week, two, or even three if you need it to declutter your kitchen and re-think the ingredients you are presently using. Follow your Ground Zero checklists to ensure your success.

PHASE 2: DETOXIFY

This phase includes week one and two. It is the most restrictive phase with regards to food ingredients. It is necessary to remove foods and hormonally reboot the body. You will not be allowed any alcohol, grains, dairy or sugar during this time. It is the hardest phase to complete however, the way you feel is well worth it! Get ready to feel energized. You can do this!

PHASE 3: DELICIOUS

This phase includes weeks three and four. You will be accustomed to making substitutions by now and well on your way to reclaiming your taste buds and enjoying all the satiating foods you are creating.

PHASE 4: DIFFERENTIATE

This phase includes weeks five through eight. You will be taught how to balance your proteins, fats and carbohydrates, plus how different people need them in different ratios. We repeat and modify recipes used in phases two and three in order to familiarize you with the recipes and increase your competence and confidence in the kitchen. You will have some freedom in this phase. Feel free to use other recipes that utilize with the ingredients listed in the "load up" and "steer clear" guidelines for the coinciding weeks.

PHASE 5: DEFY

Phase five includes weeks nine, ten, and beyond. This phase enables you to make healthy substitutions while remaking your own recipes. This lifelong way of eating will help you defy your age, as well as the unfortunate health statistics of our time.

GROUND ZERO

Our goal is to establish a kitchen of ingredients that will allow you to create a variety of meals at any time. Let's face it, a stocked, clutter-free kitchen (including the refrigerator, freezer and pantry) makes food prep easier and allows for cooking to become an enjoyable, stress-reducing daily activity.

CHECKLIST

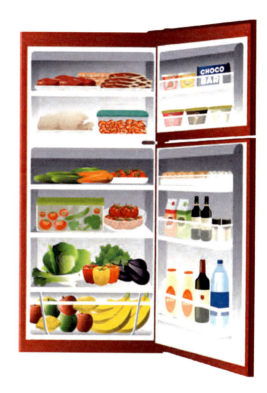

- ☑ Get Started!
- ☐ Freezer Clean Out
- ☐ Refrigerator Clean Out
- ☐ Pantry Clean Out
- ☐ Shop & Chop
- ☐ Ground Zero Tasks
    - ○ Research the shelf-life of food stored in the freezer, refrigerator and pantry
    - ○ Watch videos (www.thekeyesingredients.com)
    - ○ Make assigned recipes
        - ○ Spiced Olives
        - ○ Breading
        - ○ Carson & Isabella's Crackers
        - ○ Taco Seasoning
        - ○ Dry Rub
            - ○ Store food items for others in a solid colored Rubbermaid container
            - ○ Label foods that are off-limits

TIP!

When packaging up food use sticky notes or reminders on the containers to remind you what temperature and how long some things need to be baked for so that you dont have to go back to the recipes.

PHASE ONE

FREEZER CLEANOUT

We know this isn't the first time you have cleaned out your freezer, but have you ever cleaned it out with the intent of creating a freezer that fights disease, instead of feeding it? We want to help you construct a freezer that will provide you with the ingredients and the storage space to be successful on this journey.

LET'S GET STARTED!

- ☐ Take EVERYTHING out. Dump the ice out of the ice maker. We mean EVERYTHING!

- ☐ Wipe down all the shelves and the ice maker. White vinegar is a great natural cleaning solution.

- ☐ Throw away all items that are expired or have freezer burn.

- ☐ Make the following ingredient swaps. As far as the ingredients to toss are concerned, you can set them aside for a period of time (good option), label them to be eaten by someone who isn't on a journey towards health with you (better option), or toss them completely (best option).

Set Aside, Label or Toss	Replace with...
Baked Products	Your homemade baked goods made with better ingredients
Canned Juices	Fresh squeezed juices
Frozen Dinners	One emergency serving of fish, chicken & beef for those nights when there's "nothing for dinner"
Fruits and veggies with added sugar or sauce	Organic, no sugar added, one ingredient fruit and veggies
Sweet Treats	Frozen fruit for smoothies

FRIDGE CLEANOUT

We are working to build a refrigerator that stores ingredients in a way that the produce drawer is no longer the place where good intentions go to rot. Let's prepare our food to be eaten, not wasted!

THE GREAT FRIDGE CLEANOUT

☐ Take EVERYTHING out. Include condiments. We mean EVERYTHING!

☐ Wipe down all shelves and remove any drawers.

☐ Check the dates on all items. Throw away all items that are expired.

☐ Read the ingredients on any remaining condiments. Keep only minimal ingredient condiments without added sugar or artificial sweeteners.

☐ Make the following ingredient swaps.

Set Aside, Label or Toss	Replace with...
Breads, tortillas (packaged or fresh)	Sprouted grain bread (freezer section)
Beverages with artificial sweeteners or added sugars	Coffee, tea, sparkling water (with fresh citrus)
Commercial Dairy	Unsweetened milks (Coconut, Almond, Cashew), Pecorino Romano cheese, coconut yogurt, organic cheeses
Condiments/Dressings	Fresh herbs, mustard, organic maple syrup, organic ketchup (less sugar)
Highly processed meats (hotdogs, lunch meat, etc.)	Nitrite/nitrate-free, organic non-GMO lunch meat (use sparingly)
Jams or jelly	Whole fruit preserves (sparingly)
Juice (canned or bottles)	Whole fruit
Packaged treats/limited ingredient granola bars	Olives, fresh fruits and vegetables, pasture-raised eggs (hard boiled)

Be mindful to avoid purchasing foods with high fructose corn syrup and added sugar.

PANTRY CLEANOUT

GET READY TO TOSS!

- ☐ Take EVERYTHING out. Even what's hiding in containers. We mean EVERYTHING!
- ☐ Wipe down all shelves.
- ☐ Check the dates on everything. Throw away all items that are expired.
- ☐ Read the ingredients on any remaining products. You can set them aside (good option), label them to be eaten by someone else (better option), or get rid of them (best option).

Set Aside, Label or Toss	Replace with...
Artificial sweeteners	Coconut sugar, organic maple syrup, raw honey
Baking mixes	Almond, arrowroot, coconut flours
Boxed cereal, instant oatmeal	Granola, rolled oats, steel cut oats
Candy	Fresh fruits and berries
Canned tomatoes or pre-made/jarred spaghetti or pizza sauce	Boxed or jarred tomatoes
Flour, sugar, salt, vegetable/canola oil	Coconut oil, olive oil, coconut and almond flours, sunflower seeds, flax seeds, sesame seeds, hemp seeds, chia seeds, pumpkin seeds, black sesame seeds
Milk chocolate	72% dark chocolate or above, (the higher the percentage, the more health benefits)
Packaged snacks (pretzels, chips, popcorn, etc.)	Organic popcorn kernels, Carson's crackers, nuts (cashews, pecans, walnuts, almonds, macadamia nuts, pistachios), seeds
Pasta, oatmeal, instant potatoes	Rice, spelt pasta, shirataki noodles, sweet potatoes, white potatoes
Processed syrup	Pure organic maple syrup, raw honey

*Be mindful to avoid purchasing foods with high fructose corn syrup and added sugar.

GROCERY SHOP & CHOP

For some, it's a part of a weekly routine. For most... it is dreaded! Grocery shopping is probably one of the most procrastinated tasks that has ever existed. I want to encourage you! If you take a few simple steps, you can shop with confidence and purpose, instead of listless, hopeless, and "aw man, I forgot the..." This is the Three Step Process. We will Plan, Prepare and Provide!

PLAN

Decide which meals you and your family would like to eat for dinner this week. Once you have a list of meals, you can consult the ingredients that make up those meals and check them off on your grocery list.

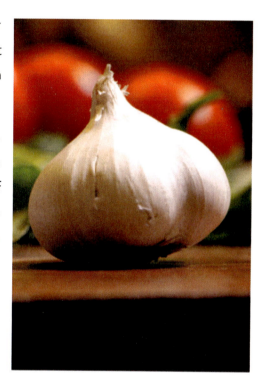

Keeping a shopping list on your device is a guaranteed way to make sure that you have your list with you at all times. There are many apps that you can download (most are free) to keep track of it for you. After making your dinner shopping list, you will have to add items that you will need for breakfast, or lunch and snacks, in addition to what you will have for dinner each evening. Meals should be planned. This does not mean you should never dine out; it simply means when you dine out, that too should be planned. Unpreparedness leaves us hungry, tired and grasping at straws for the closest and/or cheapest place to stop and "grab something."

PREPARE

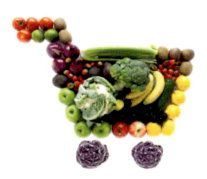

Get out that list! Shop the perimeter of the store:
- Avoid the tempting treats on the end caps
- Fill your cart with all the colors of the rainbow in the produce section.
- Avoid processed refined foods.
- Read your labels! You want to know what it means before you eat it!
- Purchase organic products when you can.
- The better quality you can buy, the better you will feel!

So you bring it all home and then what?

PROVIDE

This my grocery Chop! Put on some music, grab a knife and get to work. It is just as easy to pop the top off of ready-made, prepared whole foods as it is Pringles! They will sustain you and not cost you in the area of poor health. Invest in a few containers that will stack in your refrigerator to save space. Some items will just need to simply be transferred, and some will need to be cut or trimmed first. Transfer food to containers and into the pantry.

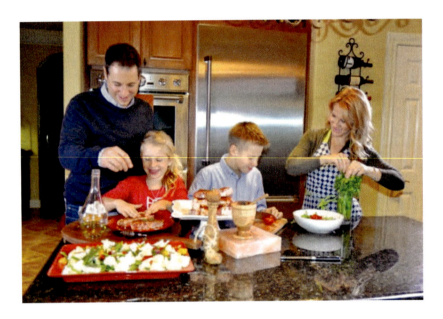

TIP!
Our pantry has our *ingredients* & our fridge has our *food*.

When you have prepared your food to be eaten and not wasted, you have provided your entire family with the opportunity to make great choices! I want you to take it one step at a time. Whether it is non-organic dairy today and organic dairy tomorrow, or "eat whatever you want" today and "I'm sorry you have to eat what I have prepared" tomorrow, **you can do this!**

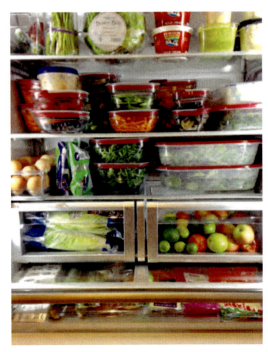

TIP!
White flour is good for one thing: Apply to a burn instantly to avoid blistering. Yellow mustard also works!

SHOP & CHOP

Preparation is the key to success! The following ingredients will be a great start to build a kitchen. These can be purchased online or from your local grocery store (many of them in the bulk bins). Quantities listed are minimum requirements for Ground Zero preparation. Feel free to purchase more to have in the future.

LET'S SHOP & CHOP!

- ☐ Almond flour 1 cup
- ☐ Chia seeds ½ cup
- ☐ Chili powder 1 cup
- ☐ Coconut flour ½ cups
- ☐ Coconut oil
- ☐ Coconut sugar ½ cups
- ☐ Cumin ¼ cup
- ☐ Dried Italian spices
- ☐ Dried onion ¼ cup
- ☐ Flax seeds 1½ cups
- ☐ Granulated garlic ¼ cup
- ☐ Hemp seeds 1 cup
- ☐ Maple syrup
- ☐ Olives 2 cups (green, black, or both)
- ☐ Olive oil
- ☐ Paprika ½ cup
- ☐ Pecorino Romano cheese 2 cups
- ☐ Pink Himalayan salt 2 cups
- ☐ Pumpkin seeds 1½ cups
- ☐ Sesame seeds 1½ cups
- ☐ Shredded, unsweetened coconut 4 cups
- ☐ Sunflower seeds 1½ cups
- ☐ Turmeric ¼ cup

Recipe	Where to Store	When to Use
Crackers	Airtight Container	Throughout the program as a snack
Grainless Breading	Freezer, Airtight Container	Weeks 3, 4, 7 & 8
Grainless Granola	Airtight Container	Throughout the program
Meat Rub	Glass Jar	Weeks 2, 3, 4, 6, 7, & 8
Olives	Glass Jar (Original Olive jar works)	Throughout the program as a snack, 4-5 at a time
Taco Seasoning	Glass Jar	Weeks 2, 3, 6 & 7

KEYES TO EATING OUT

What happens when you are invited out to eat, have a weekend getaway or need to travel for work? Before you can even speak the words "What am I supposed to eat?", your body starts freaking out, releasing one stress hormone after another! Let's put an end to that cortisol factory. I have created an emergency travel pack and restaurant guide that will save you and your lifestyle change.

FOOD CARGO

- Small cooler or bag with nuts, granola and nut butter(s). Be sure to include napkins and spoons
- Ziploc or individual packs of protein powder
- Shaker bottle
- Individual packs of organic nut butters
- Dried meat sticks (minimal ingredients)
- Nuts and seeds
- Coconut cream or coconut butter

These items will help get you through times where you need to eat something and fast food looks like the only option. If you have to skip lunch, a shake is a great meal replacement. Just remember to always replace what you have used and you will not find yourself stranded.

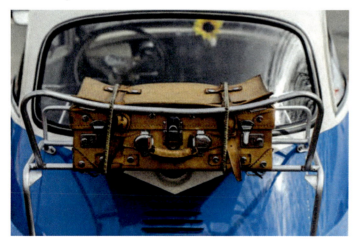

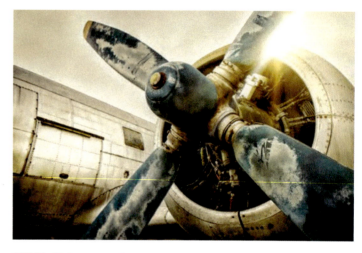

FLYING FOOD

On trips where you will be gone longer than a weekend, bring meal substitutes. Eating out adds to the inflammation levels in the body. Supplementing with a shake for even one meal is a big help. In your luggage cooler (destination dependent), pack the following items:

- Can(s) of coconut milk
- Shaker bottle
- Coconut oil or cream
- Nuts
- Crackers
- Olives
- Nut butters
- Granola/power balls
- Combine foods that have carbohydrates, fats and proteins

Note: you cannot have liquids or peanut butter in carry-on luggage

TYPES OF CUISINE & BETTER CHOICES

With any cuisine, the key is to get your macronutrients (healthy fat, protein and carbohydrates) in every meal. Be mindful of what you ate in your previous meal and what you will be eating later, if possible. This will help balance meals and satiate you for longer periods of time.

Generally, a safe meal on the go is a lean protein over a salad. This however can get old after a while so we have some suggestions.

"RULES OF TONGUE"

- Order dressing on the side. Olive oil and balsamic vinegar are preferable to a premixed dressing, which has added sugars and poor quality table salt.
- Avoid sauces, as they are salt and sugar laden.
- Pass on the complimentary breads and chips; they are appetite stimulants.
- Grilled meats over fried meats are preferable.

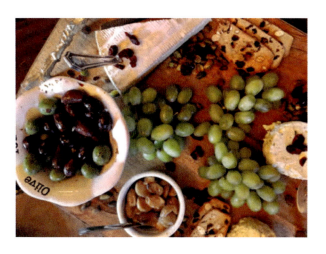

IF ENJOYING A COCKTAIL

- Avoid beer, as most are wheat-based or made with GMO corn. Choose an import if beer is your drink of choice.
- Mix spirits with soda water or fresh citrus (lime and lemon). Margarita "mix", plus tequila, equals 350 empty calories.
- Red wine, white wine or spirits on the rocks is sugar enough, as alcohol breaks down to sugar in the body.
- A healthy alcohol guideline is one to two alcoholic drinks at a time, twice per week.

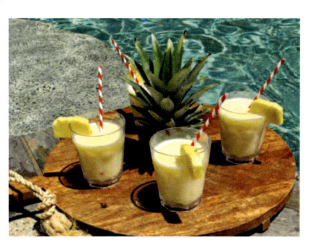

ITALIAN

- Pass on the bread. Have the server take it away, instead of agonizing over it.
- Fresh appetizers include the tomato caprese salad, grilled calamari, artichokes, and salad greens.
- A fist-sized portion of pasta is recommended. Order it on the side of chicken, veal, eggplant, or parmigiana. Perhaps ask for it to come light on cheese and add your own table side.
- Risotto is a great alternative to pasta (wheat and gluten free). Pasta mixed with vegetables is also a great balance.

MEXICAN

- Pass on the chips or restrict yourself to 6-10 (portion size).
- Most corn is GMO, especially in a restaurant.
- Choose a salad topped with chicken or beef fajita.

Note: Some restauraunts support local farms and are GMO free.

AMERICAN

- The variety in an American eatery is abundant. Consider the "rules of tongue" here.
- Avoid fried foods and order dressing on the side.
- One other thing to consider is portion sizes. Some find it helpful to order smaller portions, if available.
- Cut the meal in half and box up the other half for the next day.
- If you are dining in comfortable company, splitting a meal is a great idea.

ASIAN

- Chinese/American food is laden with corn starch-based ingredients that are very hard on your blood sugar.
- If possible, fresh is best.
- There are times where you must pick the lesser of two evils.

JAPANESE

- Sushi is made of raw fish and fresh ingredients.
- Adding ginger is a plus as it fights inflammation.
- Be mindful that fish quality is not always the best in grocery stores and/or restaurants. The mercury levels are what we want to be mindful of here.

FAST FOOD

- Although fast food places make great claims about being healthier, fast food is not an option if you want to be healthy. These foods are laced with refined sugar, table salt, poor quality meats, GMO's and chemicals.
- Brilliant marketing may have you convinced otherwise but let's face it, no one is ever going to look or feel like a million bucks eating off the dollar menu!

WEEK ONE

WHAT IS ORGANIC?

We take a "Good, Better & Best" approach to food. Conventionally grown products are good, organic products are better, and locally grown/raised food is best. For an item to be certified organic, the farmer must go through a lengthy procedure with the USDA to become certified. This ensures that his food is as safe as possible. Organic products are grown without the use of pesticides, synthetic fertilizers, sewage sludge or genetically modified organisms. Animals that produce meat, poultry, eggs and dairy products are not given antibiotics or growth hormones.

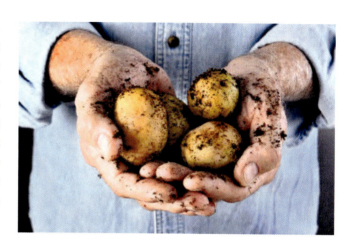

WHAT IS A GMO?

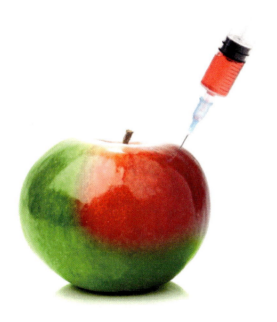

GMO's are living organisms whose genetic material has been artificially manipulated in a laboratory through genetic engineering. This relatively new science creates unstable combinations of plant, animal, bacterial and viral genes that do not occur in nature or through traditional cross-breeding methods. Virtually all GMO's are engineered to withstand direct application of herbicides and/or to produce an insecticide. Despite biotech industry promises, none of the GMO traits currently on the market increase yield, drought tolerance, enhance nutrition or any other consumer benefit. But, the GMO's have been linked with health problems and enviromental damage. They have also been banned by many developed countries, including Japan, Australia and some countries in the European Union.

- Examples of common GMO foods: corn, soy, cotton seed, alfalfa, papaya, canola and sugar beets

PHASE TWO

WEEK 1
ORGANICS / GMO'S

PRODUCE, MEAT, & DAIRY

CONVENTIONAL	ORGANIC	LOCALLY GROWN ORGANIC
GOOD	BETTER	BEST

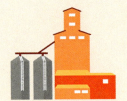

WHAT IS ORGANIC?

A FARMER MUST GO THROUGH A **LENGTHY PROCEDURE** WITH THE USDA TO BECOME **CERTIFIED**

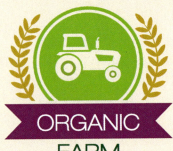
ORGANIC FARM

THIS ENSURES THAT THIS FOOD IS AS **SAFE** AS POSSIBLE

ORGANIC PRODUCTS ARE GROWN **WITHOUT** THE USE OF:

PESTICIDES
SYNTHETIC FERTILIZERS
SEWAGE SLUDGE
GENETICALLY MODIFIED ORGANISMS
IONIZING RADIATION

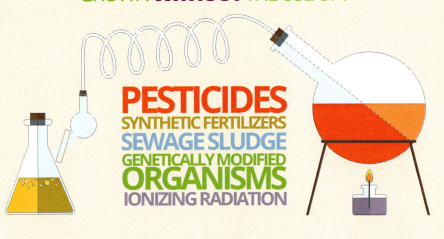

WHAT IS A GMO?

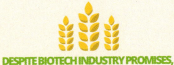

DESPITE BIOTECH INDUSTRY PROMISES, NONE OF THE GMO TRAITS CURRENTLY ON THE MARKET INCREASE YIELD, DROUGHT TOLERANCE, ENHANCE NUTRITION OR ANY OTHER CONSUMER BENEFIT, BUT THE GMO'S HAVE BEEN LINKED WITH HEALTH PROBLEMS AND ENVIRONMENTAL DAMAGE

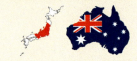

BANNED IN: JAPAN, AUSTRALIA, AND SOME COUNTRIES IN THE EUROPEAN UNION

GMO'S ARE LIVING ORGANISMS WHOSE GENETIC MATERIAL HAS BEEN **ARTIFICIALLY MANIPULATED** IN A LABORATORY THROUGH GENETIC ENGINEERING

THIS RELATIVELY NEW SCIENCE CREATES UNSTABLE COMBINATIONS OF PLANT, ANIMAL, BACTERIAL AND VIRAL GENES THAT DO NOT OCCUR IN NATURE OR THROUGH TRADITIONAL CROSSBREEDING METHODS

EXAMPLES: CORN, SOY, COTTON SEED, ALFALFA, PAPAYA, CANOLA AND SUGAR BEETS

LOAD UP! WEEK ONE

MEATS
(Pasture raised or organic is best)
beef, bison, lamb

POULTRY
(Pasture raised or organic is best)
chicken, duck, turkey, cornish game hens

FISH
(Wild caught best)
Cod, Grouper, Mahi Mahi, Snapper, Tuna, Sole Orange Roughy, Haddock, Salmon, Trout

EGGS
(Pasture raised hens are best)
chicken eggs, duck eggs

DAIRY
(Should be EXTREMELY limited, small portions, infrequently)
Pecorino Romano (sheep's milk cheese), goat or sheep milk products only

FATS & OILS
avocado, grass-fed butter, coconut oil, olive oil, organic ghee

VEGETABLES
(organic, fresh or frozen)
artichoke, asparagus, broccoli, brussels sprouts, cabbage, carrots, cauliflower, chard, celery, cucumber, eggplant, escarole, garlic, green beans, green onions, leeks, lettuce, mushrooms, olives, onion, peas, pumpkin, turnip, rutabaga, squash, tomato

HERBS
(organic, fresh or frozen)
basil, parsley, dill, oregano, cilantro, rosemary, thyme, sage, mint

BEANS & LEGUMES
omit all

NUTS & SEEDS
(unprocessed/unsalted)
almonds, cashews, chia, coconut, flaxseed, hazelnut, hempseed, macadamia, pecans, pumpkin, sunflower, walnuts, nuts/seed butters

SPICES
(suggested, but not limited to)
basil, cayenne pepper, Celtic sea salt, cumin, cinnamon, cracked pepper, garlic, ginger, Himalayan salt, rosemary, thyme, turmeric, paprika, Italian seasoning, onion, garlic, vanilla

FRUITS
lemons, limes

BEVERAGES
water, water, water (for detoxification purposes), carbonated water (limited), Kombucha (fermented green tea, read label for sugar content), herbal teas, organic coffee, vegetable juice, coconut water, unsweetened nut milks (coconut, almond, cashew)

STEER CLEAR! WEEK ONE

MEATS
pork, breaded/fried meats

POULTRY
breaded/fried poultry

FISH
shellfish, breaded/fried fish

EGGS
imitation eggs, Egg Beaters

DAIRY
avoid all cow's milk products.

FATS & OILS
canola oil (GMO), corn oil, lard, safflower oil, margarine, soybean oil, cottonseed oil, hydrogenated or partially hydrogenated oils

VEGETABLES
white potatoes, corn, sweet potato

BEANS & LEGUMES
soy beans, garbanzo beans, white beans, black beans, tofu, navy beans, kidney beans, lentils

NUTS & SEEDS
peanuts (they are a legume)

CONDIMENTS/SPICES
any that contain added sugar (read the label)

FRUITS
avoid all (see "Eat This! Week One")

BEVERAGES
alcoholic, sodas (diet and regular), energy drinks

GRAINS
oats, breads, pastas, rice, cereal, pastries, baked goods (anything with flour)

SWEETENERS
sugar, high fructose corn syrup, sugar alcohol, xylitol, sorbitol, all artificial sweeteners

WEEK ONE MEALS

BREAKFAST

These are suggested breakfast items. Breakfast may be substituted with a shake, balanced in proteins, fats and carbs.

EGGS: scrambled, boiled, fried, omelette (add herbs, onions, tomatoes, greens and/or avocado)

FRITTATA MUFFIN

GRAINLESS GRANOLA (1/4-1/3 cup)

CHIA PUDDING (1/4-1/2 cup)

LUNCH

Lunches should be purposeful leftovers from dinner the night before. Leftovers can be accompanied by:

SOUP

RAW OR COOKED VEGETABLES

BOILED EGG

OLIVES (3-5)

FRESH MIXED GREENS (1/4-1/2 cup)

DINNER

You may eat the meals in the order you choose.

LEMON CHICKEN with Ceaser salad

VEGETABLE SPAGHETTI & BOLOGNESE SAUCE

PAPA'S CHICKEN SOUP with salad

5 HOUR STEW with salad (make the day before)

SESAME CRUSTED SALMON with veggie medley

PURPOSEFUL LEFTOVERS

DINE OUT to challenge yourself to make great choices.

SNACKS

These are approved snacks that are optional. Be mindful to combine a protein, a fat and a carbohydrate with snack options.

- CARSON'S CRACKERS
- HARD BOILED EGGS
- SICILIAN SPICED OLIVES
- PECORINO ROMANO CHEESE
- NUTS/NUT BUTTER*
- UNSALTED SEEDS*
- PROTEIN SHAKE WITH NUT MILK
- GRANOLA/POWER BALLS
- AVOCADO/VEGGIES

*Read and understand your labels. Be mindful of unhealthy salt & oils.

Portions

 complex carbs
 protein
 healthy fat
 snack

WEEK ONE GROCERIES

This list includes items you will use for dinner and potentially lunches the next day. **Be sure to add in fresh items to make breakfasts and prepare snacks.** Organic or local fresh farm raised items are preferred.

Double check your stock pantry list to make sure you have the essentials.

MEATS

Unless otherwise specified, the recommended serving size will depend on the number of portions. The recommended amount of meat/fish per serving is 1/2 pound.

- [ ] 1 whole chicken (for soup)
- [ ] 3-4 pounds of steak/stewing beef (for stew)
- [ ] 1-2 pounds of ground meat (for meat sauce)
- [ ] wild caught salmon filet (or chicken)
- [ ] chicken breasts
  (for marinated chicken on Ceasar salad)

AISLE

- [ ] Tobasco
- [ ] Worcestershire
- [ ] Dijon mustard
- [ ] red wine vinegar
- [ ] red wine
- [ ] anchovy paste (optional)
- [ ] coconut/olive oil
- [ ] dried Italian spices
- [ ] Himalayan salt
- [ ] beef broth
- [ ] 5-24 oz jars/boxes of crushed/diced tomatoes
  (5 lbs of fresh tomatoes can be used)

REFRIGERATED SECTION

- [ ] 1-2 dozen eggs
- [ ] coconut/almond milk (unsweetened)
- [ ] Pecorino Romano Cheese (whole or grated)

PRODUCE

- [ ] 2 bags of carrots (fresh or frozen)
- [ ] onions (4-6 fresh or 3 bags frozen)
- [ ] 2 bunches of celery (pre-chopped optional)
- [ ] 1 red bell pepper (for medley)
- [ ] butternut squash (1 fresh or 2 bags frozen)
- [ ] turnip greens (1-2 fresh or 1 bag frozen)
- [ ] spaghetti squash OR zucchini (1 per person)
- [ ] bunch asparagus (for medley)
- [ ] zucchini (for medley)
- [ ] cauliflower (pre-cut for medley) or 1 head
- [ ] 3-4 lemons or bottled lemon juice
- [ ] 1 package of fresh dill (to garnish stew)
- [ ] basil (fresh or frozen) (for Bolognese sauce)
- [ ] 1 bunch of fresh parsley (for soup)
- [ ] 1 bunch of Swiss chard (for Bolognese)
- [ ] greens for salads (arugula, spinach, kale, etc.)
- [ ] garlic (1-2 heads)

This list includes items you will need for dinners and most lunches. Be sure to add items you will need for breakfasts and other members of your household.

WEEK TWO

SUGARS & SUGAR SUBSTITUTES

THE EFFECTS OF SUGAR ON YOUR BODY

Your body can only properly metabolize about six teaspoons of sugar (and all other processed fructose, high fructose corn syrup, etc.) per day. The average American consumes almost 22 tablespoons per day. When your body is unable to process that, it turns into body fat and leads to Type 2 diabetes, cardiovascular disease, hypertension, dementia and cancer. Four grams of sugar is the equivalent to one teaspoon. It is highly recommended that you limit sugar (including that from natural sources like fruit, maple syrup, honey, etc.) to 25 grams (6 teaspoons) a day. If you are in Metabolic Syndrome or have Insulin Resistance, it is recommended to be cut to less than 15 grams per day until you have normalized your blood sugar and have it under good control.

ASPARTAME

Often branded Equal, Aspartame is a common substance found in many "diet" and sugar-free foods. It is marketed as a sugar-free sweetener. It is made up of aspartic acid and phenylalanine. The later has been synthetically altered to carry a methyl group, which is responsible for the sweet taste. The bond, called methyl ester, allows the methyl group on the phenylalanine to break off and form mathanol. This same substance is found in fruit, but is bonded to pectin so it allows it to be safely passed through your digestive tract. In aspartame, however, methanol is not bonded so it is not allowed to eliminate. Once it is inside your body, it is converted by ADH enzymes into formaldehyde. It is known to cause birth defects, epilepsy, cancer, and emotional disorders.

PHASE TWO

WEEK TWO

SUGARS & SUGAR SUBSTITUTES (CONTINUED)

SACCHARIN

Often branded Sweet N Low, Saccharin is the first artificial sweetener and was discovered in 1879 when Constantin Fahlberg was working on creating a coal-tar derivative at Johns Hopkins University. He licked the remaining substance on his arms and noticed that it had a sweet aftertaste. At that point saccharin was born. It is known to be 300 times sweeter than sugar and has a metallic aftertaste. It was also the first artuficial sweetener to carry a label of being a known carcinogen. The FDA has since removed this label, but the formula for saccharin has not changed.

SUCRALOSE

Often branded Splenda, Sucralose is a substance that has attempted to become the "safe" alternative to aspartame. This is definitely not the case. Sucralose has been known to cause toxicity, DNA damage and increased carcinogenic potential when it is used in cooking. When heated, it releases chloropropanols, which belong to a class of toxins known as dioxins. Dioxin is a waste product of incineration, smelting, chlorine bleaching and pesticide manufacturing, and its well documented health effects include cancer and endocrine disruption. Sucralose is also dangerous for diabetics because it is known to alter both insulin and the insulin secretion rate.

At the end of the day, sugar is still sugar and excess sugar is stored as fat. If your goal is to lose weight, limit your fructose to 15 grams a day. If maintaining a healthy weight limit your fructose to 25 grams a day.

Approximate Sugar/Fructrose Content in Common Fruits in grams per 1 Cup serving

Fruit	Grams	Fruit	Grams
Lemon/Lime	0.5	Pears	16
Grapefruit	16	Oranges	17
Blueberries	7	Peaches	13
Blackberries	7	Bananas	18
Raspberries	3	Grapes	23
Strawberries	7	Pineapple	16
Melons	12	Raisins	86
Apples	19		

Avoid dried fruit or use sparingly.

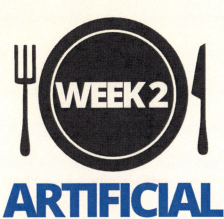

WEEK 2
ARTIFICIAL SWEETENER

YOUR LIVER CAN ONLY PROPERLY METABOLIZE ABOUT
6 TEASPOONS OF SUGAR PER DAY

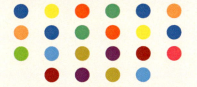

THE AVERAGE AMERICAN CONSUMES
ALMOST 22 TEASPOONS A DAY

WHEN YOUR BODY IS UNABLE TO PROCESS THAT, IT TURNS INTO BODY FAT AND LEADS TO
**TYPE 2 DIABETES
CARDIOVASCULAR DISEASE
HYPERTENSION
DEMENTIA
CANCER**

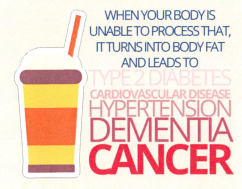

IT IS HIGHLY RECOMMENDED THAT YOU LIMIT SUGAR (INCLUDING THAT FROM NATURAL SOURCES LIKE FRUIT, MAPLE SYRUP, HONEY, ETC) TO 6 TEASPOONS A DAY

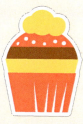

(IF YOU ARE IN METABOLIC SYNDROME OR HAVE INSULIN RESISTANCE ISSUES, IT IS RECOMMENDED TO BE CUT TO LESS THAN 15 GRAMS PER DAY UNTIL YOU HAVE NORMALIZED THOSE LEVELS)

COMMON SUBSTANCE FOUND IN MANY "DIET" AND SUGAR-FREE FOODS. IT IS MARKETED AS A SUGAR FREE SWEETENER. IT IS MADE UP OF ASPARTIC ACID AND PHENYLALANINE

ONCE IT IS INSIDE YOUR BODY, IT IS CONVERTED BY ADH ENZYMES INTO FORMALDEHYDE. IT IS KNOWN TO CAUSE:
**BIRTH DEFECTS
EPILEPSY
CANCER
EMOTIONAL DISORDERS**

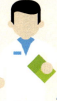

DISCOVERED IN 1879 WHEN CONSTANTIN FAHLBERG WAS WORKING ON CREATING A COAL-TAR DERIVATIVE AT JOHNS HOPKINS UNIVERSITY. HE LICKED THE REMAINING SUBSTANCE ON HIS ARMS AND NOTICED THAT IT HAD A SWEET AFTERTASTE AND SACCHARIN WAS BORN

300X SWEETER THAN SUGAR

SUCRALOSE IS A SUBSTANCE THAT HAS ATTEMPTED TO BECOME THE "SAFE" ALTERNATIVE TO ASPARTAME
THIS IS DEFINITELY NOT THE CASE

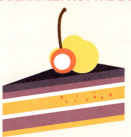

SUCRALOSE HAS BEEN KNOWN TO CAUSE **TOXICITY, DNA DAMAGE AND INCREASED CARCINOGENIC POTENTIAL** WHEN IT IS USED IN COOKING

ASPARTAME
(OFTEN BRANDED EQUAL)

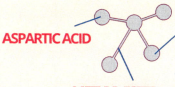

ASPARTIC ACID

PHENYLALANINE SYNTHETICALLY ALTERED TO CARRY A METHYL GROUP, WHICH IS RESPONSIBLE FOR THE SWEET TASTE

METHYL ESTER ALLOWS THE METHYL GROUP ON THE PHENYLALANINE TO BREAK OFF AND FORM METHANOL

METHANOL IS FOUND IN FRUIT, BUT IS BONDED TO PECTIN SO IT ALLOWS IT TO BE SAFELY PASSED THROUGH YOUR DIGESTIVE TRACT

IN ASPARTAME, METHANOL IS NOT BONDED SO IT IS NOT ALLOWED TO ELIMINATE

SACCHARIN
(OFTEN BRANDED SWEET N' LOW)

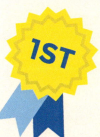

1ST ARTIFICIAL SWEETENER

1ST ARTIFICIAL SWEETENER TO CARRY A LABEL OF BEING A **KNOWN CARCINOGEN** (THE FDA HAS SINCE REMOVED THIS LABEL, BUT THE FORMULA FOR SACCHARIN HAS NOT CHANGED)

SUCRALOSE
(OFTEN BRANDED SPLENDA)

WHEN HEATED, IT RELEASES **CHLOROPROPANOLS**, WHICH BELONG TO A CLASS OF TOXINS KNOWN AS **DIOXINS**. DIOXIN IS A WASTE PRODUCT OF INCINERATION, SMELTING, CHLORINE BLEACHING, AND PESTICIDE MANUFACTURING, AND **ITS WELL-DOCUMENTED HEALTH EFFECTS INCLUDE CANCER AND ENDOCRINE DISRUPTION**

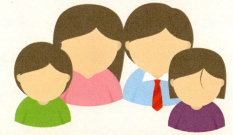

SUCRALOSE IS ALSO DANGEROUS FOR **DIABETICS** BECAUSE IT IS KNOWN TO ALTER BOTH INSULIN AND THE INSULIN SECRETION RATE

LOAD UP! WEEK TWO

MEATS
(Pasture raised or organic is best)
beef, bison, lamb

POULTRY
(Pasture raised or organic is best)
chicken, duck, turkey, cornish game hens

FISH
(Wild caught best)
Cod, Grouper, Mahi Mahi, Snapper, Tuna, Sole Orange Roughy, Haddock, Salmon, Trout

EGGS
(Pasture raised hens are best)
chicken eggs, duck eggs

DAIRY
(Should be EXTREMELY limited, small portions, infrequently)
Pecorino Romano (sheep's milk cheese), goat or sheep milk products

FATS & OILS
avocado, grass-fed butter, coconut oil, olive oil, organic ghee

VEGETABLES
(organic, fresh or frozen) not limited to
artichoke, asparagus, broccoli, brussels sprouts, cabbage, carrots, cauliflower, chard, celery, cucumber, eggplant, escarole, garlic, green onions, leeks, lettuce, mushrooms, olives, onion, peas, turnip, rutabaga, squash, pumpkin

HERBS
(organic, fresh or frozen)
basil, parsley, dill, oregano, cilantro, rosemary, thyme, sage, mint

BEANS & LEGUMES
omit all

NUTS & SEEDS
(unprocessed/unsalted)
almonds, cashews, chia, coconut, flaxseed, hazelnut, hempseed, macadamia, pecans, pumpkin, sunflower, walnuts, nuts/seed butters

SPICES
(suggested but not limited to)
basil, Celtic sea salt, cumin, cinnamon, cracked pepper, ginger, Himalayan salt, rosemary, thyme, turmeric, paprika, Italian seasoning, onion, garlic, vanilla

FRUITS
lemons, limes, berries

BEVERAGES
water, water, water (for detoxification purposes), carbonated water (limited), Kombucha (fermented green tea, read label for sugar content), herbal teas, organic coffee, vegetable juice, coconut water, coconut milk

STEER CLEAR! WEEK TWO

MEATS
pork, breaded/fried meats

POULTRY
breaded/fried poultry

FISH
shellfish, breaded/fried fish

EGGS
imitation eggs, Egg Beaters

DAIRY
avoid all cow's milk products

FATS & OILS
canola oil (GMO), corn oil, lard, safflower oil, margarine, soybean oil, cottonseed oil, hydrogenated or partially hydrogenated oils

VEGETABLES
white potatoes, corn, sweet potato

BEANS & LEGUMES
soy beans, garbanzo beans, white beans, black beans, tofu, navy beans, kidney beans, lentils

NUTS & SEEDS
peanuts

CONDIMENTS/SPICES
any that contain added sugar (read the label)

FRUITS
avoid most (see "Eat This! Week Two")

BEVERAGES
caffinated, alcoholic, sodas (diet and regular), energy drinks

GRAINS
oats, breads, pastas, rice, cereal, pastries, baked goods (anything with flour)

SWEETENERS
sugar, high fructose corn syrup, sugar alcohol, xylitol, sorbitol, all artificial sweeteners

WEEK TWO MEALS

BREAKFAST

These are suggested breakfast items. Breakfast may be substituted with a shake, balanced in proteins, fats, and carbs.

EGGS: scrambled, boiled, fried, omelette (add herbs, onions, tomatoes, greens and/or avocado)

FRITTATA MUFFIN

GRAINLESS GRANOLA (1/4-1/3 cup)

CHIA PUDDING (1/4-1/2 cup)

DINNER

You may eat the meals in the order you choose.

TACO SALAD (beef OR chicken) with cilantro lime dressing. Omit beans

PAPA'S MINESTRONE with salad

SPICED DRY RUB CHICKEN with garden salad (freeze carcass for week four)

ALMOND CRUSTED FISH with vegetable medley

DRY RUBBED STEAK & CAULIFLOWER MASH with spinach

PURPOSEFUL LEFTOVERS

DINE OUT to challenge yourself to make great choices.

LUNCH

Lunches should be purposeful leftovers from dinner the night before. Leftovers can be accompanied by:

SOUP

RAW OR COOKED VEGETABLES

BOILED EGG

OLIVES (3-5)

FRESH MIXED GREENS topped with protein

SNACKS

These are approved snacks that are optional. Be mindful to combine a protein, a fat and a carbohydrate with snack options.

- CARSON'S CRACKERS
- HARD BOILED EGGS
- SICILIAN SPICED OLIVES
- PECORINO ROMANO CHEESE
- NUTS/NUT BUTTER
- UNSALTED SEEDS
- PROTEIN SHAKE WITH NUT MILK
- GRANOLA/POWER BALLS
- AVOCADO/ VEGGIES

Read and understand your labels. Be mindful of unhealthy salt & oils.

Portions

complex carbs   protein   healthy fat   snack

WEEK TWO GROCERIES

This list includes items you will use for dinner and potentially lunches the next day. Be sure to add in fresh items to make breakfasts and prepare snacks. Organic or local fresh farm raised items are preferred.

Double check your stock pantry list to make sure you have the essentials. If you have already made your meat rub, taco seasoning and breading, the "aisle" ingredients will be minimal. Spices can be purchased in larger quantities online. (*marks the ingredients you will not need.)

MEATS

Unless otherwise specified, the recommended serving size will depend on the number of portions. The recommended amount of meat/fish per serving is 1/2 pound.

- [ ] whole chicken (for spice rubbed chicken)
- [ ] 2 pounds of ground beef or chicken (taco salad)
- [ ] 1 pound of ground beef (meat option in minestrone)
- [ ] white fish (chicken may be substituted)
- [ ] grass fed-steaks (for spiced dry rubbed steak)

REFRIGERATED SECTION

- [ ] eggs for breakfast & hard boiled (for snacks/taco salad)
- [ ] coconut milk (unsweetened)
- [ ] coconut yogurt (plain/unsweetened; no more than 1-2 grams of sugar)
- [ ] Pecorino Romano cheese 3 cups** (check local wholesale clubs for value; for breading and as a soup topper)

AISLE

- [ ] coconut and/or olive oil
- [ ] dried Italian herbs**
- [ ] Himalayan salt*
- [ ] cumin*
- [ ] granulated garlic*
- [ ] flax seeds*
- [ ] sesame seeds*
- [ ] hemp seeds/hearts*
- [ ] paprika*
- [ ] chili powder*
- [ ] slivered almonds**
- [ ] dried onion*
- [ ] almond flour**
- [ ] coconut flour**
- [ ] 2 cups red wine (for cooking)
- [ ] organic coffee grounds (steak dry rub optional)

*Omit these ingredients if dry rub and taco seasoning is already prepped

**Omit these ingredients if breading is already prepped

This list includes items you will need for dinners and most lunches. Be sure to add items you will need for breakfasts and other members of your household.

WEEK TWO GROCERIES

PRODUCE

- [ ] carrots (1 bag fresh for chicken, 1 bag (pre-cut coins) frozen for soup)
- [ ] 1 bag of frozen peas (for minestrone soup; frozen peas and carrots are available together)
- [ ] onions (3-4 fresh or 2 bags of pre-cut frozen for soup and taco salad)
- [ ] 1 bunch fresh cilantro (taco salad dressing)
- [ ] 1 head of iceberg lettuce (taco salad)
- [ ] 1 purple onion (available pre-chopped)
- [ ] 1 bunch of celery (pre-chopped optional)
- [ ] collard greens 1 bunch fresh or 1 bag frozen (for minestrone)
- [ ] 1-2 red bell peppers (for vegetable medley and taco salad)
- [ ] 1 jalapeño pepper (for salad dressing - omit if you do not like spicy)
- [ ] butternut squash (purchase pre-chopped or frozen)
- [ ] 1 bunch of asparagus (for vegetable medley)
- [ ] 1 zucchini (for vegetable medley)
- [ ] cauliflower for vegetable medley (pre-cut or 1 head)
- [ ] 1 bag frozen, pre-cut or head of cauliflower (for cauliflower mash)
- [ ] 1-2 bags of spinach (fresh or frozen)
- [ ] 2-3 limes or bottled lime juice
- [ ] basil fresh or frozen cubes
- [ ] 1 bunch of fresh parsley
- [ ] 2-3 heads of fresh garlic, jarred or frozen
- [ ] lettuce for salads (romaine, iceberg, spinach, kale, arugula, mixed greens)
- [ ] 1 cucumber (taco salad)
- [ ] 2-3 avocados (taco salad/taco salad dressing)
- [ ] 2 pounds of fresh tomatoes or jarred/boxed diced (for minestrone)
- [ ] 1 package of grape tomatoes (for taco salad)
- [ ] salad toppers (fresh veggies you prefer)
- [ ] nuts and seeds (pumpkin seeds top the taco salad for crunch)

WEEK THREE

DAIRY

CONVENTIONAL DAIRY

The majority of dairy sold in stores today have multiple issues that can affect your health. Many dairy cows are fed GMO feed that may also contain antibiotics and growth hormones (rBST). These animals are often raised in inhumane conditions. All these factors affect the quality of the milk produced. To further complicate the matter, the milk is pasteurized. The pasteurization process was developed to kill harmful bacteria in the milk. During pasteurization milk is heated to high temperatures, killing all good and bad bacteria, and unfortunately destroys essential nutrients and vitamins, denaturing proteins. Have you ever wondered why the lunch box size milks are in the aisle? In Europe you will find pasteurized dairy unrefrigerated. In the United States dairy is refrigerated simply to make us feel better about buying it. It has nothing to do with maintaining freshness. Pasteurized products will keep in or out of the refrigerator until opened. Once opened and exposed to airborne bacteria and oxygen they are more prone to perish. Most commercial dairy cows are of the Holstein breed which produce milk containing the A1 Casein protein. This casein protein is highly inflammatory and the reason why so many people feel stuffy and have runny nose is after consuming commercial dairy.

RAW DAIRY

Raw milk does not undergo the pasteurization process. This maintains the integrity of proteins, nutrients, vitamins and good bacteria. This was the only dairy available prior to pasteurization. When animals are healthy and milk is collected in a sanitary environment, the nutrient content is much greater. Raw dairy is known to have higher levels of magnesium, potassium, calcium and vitamin D. Dairy is not essential for the human diet. Many make the argument that humans are the only ones to consume the milk of another animal. The majority of raw milk today comes from Jersey cows. This breed produces milk containing the A2 casein protein which is far less inflammatory and better digested. Goat and sheep milk also contain the A2 Casein protein. This is why some people can tolerate goat or sheep dairy products over cows milk products.

PHASE THREE

WEEK THREE

ORGANIC DAIRY

Organic dairy is a better option than conventional dairy and is much more readily available than raw dairy. Organic dairy comes from cows that have been regulated in the way they are fed and raised. They must be given organic feed and allowed access to the outdoors and a certain amount of grazing room. They are also raised without the use of antibiotics and artificial growth hormones. These cows produce milk that is higher in protein and Omega 3's due to their better living conditions.

DAIRY ALTERNATIVES

GOAT/SHEEP CHEESE & MILK

Sheep cheese is sweeter than cows cheese and contains higher levels of protein and calcium. It is richer in beneficial fatty acids, specifically omega-3's and conjugated linoleic acid. These fatty acids are known to help lower cholesterol and lower cancer risks. They also aid in maintaining a healthy weight. The short and medium chain fatty acids in this cheese make it more gentle on your digestive system. Similarly goats cheese is more readily digestible than cows dairy. It contains smaller fat globules. Goats cheese has a very distinct flavor that some love and others find pungent. Both goat and sheep's milk are less inflammatory and do not affect the mucosal membranes like regular commercial dairy.

COCONUT PRODUCTS

Coconut milk is a milk alternative that contains many of the same nutritional benefits as raw milk. It is not actually milk, but the water from the inside of the coconut, combined with the meat from the fruit to make a creamy milk-like substance with a sweet taste. Coconut milk contains fatty acids that are known to lower cholesterol levels and improve blood sugar. It also helps build muscles and lose fat. Coconut products also nourish the digestive lining due to electrolytes and healthy fat, reducing constipation and improving digestion.

NUT MILK

Milk made from nuts (coconut, almond, cashew, etc.) is another naturally lactose free, dairy free milk alternative . Nut milks are often times sweetened, so make sure you are purchasing **unsweetened** nut milks.

WEEK 3
DAIRY

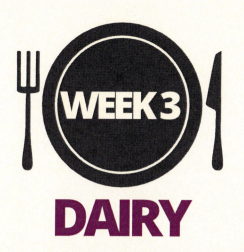

MOST DAIRY SOLD IN OUR STORES TODAY HAS MULTIPLE STRIKES AGAINST IT AS FAR AS BECOMING FUEL FOR YOUR BODY

CONVENTIONAL

COMES FROM COWS THAT HAVE BEEN TREATED WITH **ANTIBIOTICS AND GROWTH HORMONES** THEY ARE OFTEN RAISED IN INHUMANE CONDITIONS AS WELL

PASTEURIZATION HEATS MILK TO THE POINT THAT IT KILLS BACTERIA AND THEN BRINGS IT BACK TO A COOL TEMPERATURE. **IT ALSO KILLS MOST OF THE VALUABLE VITAMINS AND MINERALS IN THE PROCESS.** A FEW ARE THEN ARTIFICIALLY PUT BACK IN

GOOD

ORGANIC

MUCH MORE READILY AVAILABLE THAN RAW DAIRY
COMES FROM COWS THAT HAVE BEEN REGULATED IN THE WAY THEY ARE FED AND RAISED. THEY MUST BE GIVEN **ORGANIC FEED** AND ALLOWED ACCESS TO THE OUTDOORS AND A CERTAIN AMOUNT OF GRAZING ROOM

THEY ARE ALSO RAISED WITHOUT THE USE OF **ANTIBIOTICS**
ARTIFICIAL GROWTH HORMONES
THESE COWS PRODUCE MILK THAT IS HIGHER IN PROTEIN AND OMEGA 3'S DUE TO THEIR BETTER LIVING CONDITIONS

BETTER

RAW

COMES DIRECTLY FROM THE ANIMAL AND **SKIPS** THE **PASTEURIZATION PROCESS** ABLE TO KEEP MANY OF ITS VITAL NUTRIENTS. RAW MILK IS HIGH IN OMEGA 3'S, CALCIUM, MAGNESIUM AND POTASSIUM

HAS NATURALLY OCCURRING **PROBIOTICS** AND **HEALTHY FATS** THAT ARE BENEFICIAL FOR BOTH GUT AND SKIN HEALTH

BEST

SHEEP CHEESE

MORE **PROTEIN, CALCIUM, AND SWEETER** THAN COWS MILK CHEESE

RICH IN BENEFICIAL FATTY ACIDS, SPECIFICALLY **OMEGA-3 AND CONJUGATED LINOLEIC ACID**

REDUCES CHOLESTEROL, LOWER CANCER RISKS AND AID IN WEIGHT LOSS

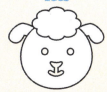

SHORT AND MEDIUM CHAIN FATTY ACIDS MAKE IT **GENTLER ON YOUR DIGESTIVE SYSTEM** AS WELL

COCONUT PRODUCTS

WATER FROM THE INSIDE OF THE COCONUT COMBINED WITH MEAT FROM THE FRUIT AND MAKES A CREAMY SWEET MILK LIKE SUBSTANCE
MANY OF THE SAME NUTRITIONAL BENEFITS AS RAW MILK

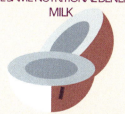

CONTAINS FATTY ACIDS THAT ARE KNOWN TO:
LOWER CHOLESTEROL LEVELS
IMPROVE BLOOD SUGAR **LOSE FAT** BUILD MUSCLES
NOURISHES THE DIGESTIVE LINING DUE TO ELECTROLYTES AND HEALTHY FAT REDUCING CONSTIPATION AND IMPROVING DIGESTION

NUT MILKS

NATURALLY **LACTOSE FREE, DAIRY FREE**, MILK ALTERNATIVE
LOW IN SATURATE FAT AND CHOLESTEROL

GOOD SOURCE OF VITAMIN **A** AND **D**

NUT MILKS INCLUDE BUT ARE NOT LIMITED TO: ALMOND, COCONUT, AND CASHEW

LOAD UP! WEEK THREE

Please continue to load up on the same ingredients that were in your Weeks 1 & 2. Use moderation in continuing to introduce new items. Items in green have been reintroduced into your diet. Please pay attention and journal how you feel after eating them.

MEATS
(Pasture raised or organic is best)
beef, bison, lamb

POULTRY
(Pasture raised or organic is best)
chicken, duck, turkey, cornish game hens

FISH
(Wild caught is best)
Cod, Grouper, Mahi Mahi, Snapper, Tuna, Sole Orange Roughy, Haddock, Salmon, Trout

EGGS
(Pasture raised hens are best)
chicken eggs, duck eggs

DAIRY
goat's or sheep milk products, raw or organic cream (for coffee), raw or organic milk (in small amounts)

FATS & OILS
avocado, grass-fed butter, coconut oil, olive oil, organic ghee

VEGETABLES
(organic, fresh or frozen) ALL vegetables, white potatoes, corn (non GMO), sweet potatoes (keep to fist sized portions)

SWEETENERS
coconut sugar, honey, maple syrup, stevia

BEANS & LEGUMES
black beans, navy beans, white beans, kidney beans, garbanzo beans (portion fist sized)

NUTS & SEEDS
(unprocessed/raw)
almonds, cashews, chia, coconut, flaxseed, hazelnut, hempseed, macadamia, pecans, pumpkin, sunflower, walnuts, nuts/seed butters

SPICES
(suggested, but not limited to)
basil, Celtic sea salt, cumin, cinnamon, cracked pepper, ginger, Himalayan salt, rosemary, thyme, turmeric, paprika, Italian seasoning, onion, garlic, vanilla, anything that doesn't contain sugar

FRUITS
ALL fruits, be mindful of how many grams of natural sugar

BEVERAGES
an occasional alcoholic beverage is permitted (avoiding is best)

HERBS
(organic, fresh or frozen) basil, parsley, dill, oregano, cilantro, sage rosemary, mint

STEER CLEAR! WEEK THREE

MEATS
pork

FISH
shellfish

EGGS
imitation eggs, Egg Beaters

DAIRY
soy milk (GMO)

FATS & OILS
canola oil (GMO), corn oil, lard, safflower oil, margarine, soybean oil, cottonseed oil, hydrogenated or partially hydrogenated oils

BEANS & LEGUMES
soy beans, tofu

NUTS & SEEDS
dry, roasted in oil, honey roasted

CONDIMENTS/SPICES
any that contain added sugar (read the label)

FRUITS
See page 37 for guide

BEVERAGES
alcoholic (limited), ABSOLUTELY NO soda

GRAINS
breads, pastas, rice, cereal, pastries, baked goods (anything with flour)

SWEETENERS
sugar, high fructose corn syrup, sugar alcohol, xylitol, sorbitol, all artificial sweeteners

WEEK THREE MEALS

BREAKFAST

These are suggested breakfast items. Breakfast may be substituted with a shake, balanced in proteins, fats and carbs.

EGGS: scrambled, boiled, fried, omelette (add herbs, onions, tomatoes, greens and/or avocado)

FRITTATA MUFFIN

GRAINLESS GRANOLA (1/4-1/3 cup)

SHAKE can be used as a meal replacement

CHIA PUDDING (1/4-1/2 cup)

EGGS FOR A CROWD

DINNER

You may eat the meals in the order you choose.

LENTIL SOUP with salad

BEEF BURGERS WITH BUTTERY GREEN BEANS and salad

CHICKEN/FISH recipe of your choice and **VEGETABLE MEDLEY** with salad

EGG PARMIGIANA & VEGETABLE PASTA with salad

WHITE BEAN CHICKEN CHILI with salad

PURPOSEFUL LEFTOVERS

DINE OUT to challenge yourself to make great choices.

LUNCH

Lunches should be purposeful leftovers from dinner the night before. Leftovers can be accompanied by:

SOUP

RAW OR COOKED VEGETABLES

BOILED EGG

OLIVES (3-5)

GOAT OR SHEEP MILK CHEESE small amount

FRESH MIXED GREENS topped with protein

SNACKS

These are approved snacks that are optional. Be mindful to combine a protein, a fat and a carbohydrate with snack options.

- CARSON'S CRACKERS
- HARD BOILED EGGS
- SICILIAN SPICED OLIVES
- PECORINO ROMANO CHEESE
- NUTS/NUT BUTTER
- UNSALTED SEEDS
- PROTEIN SHAKE WITH COCONUT MILK
- GRANOLA/POWER BALLS
- AVOCADO/WHOLE FRUIT/ VEGGIES

Read and understand your labels. Be mindful of unhealthy salt & oils.

 Portions complex carbs protein healthy fat snack

WEEK THREE GROCERIES

This list includes items you will use for dinner and potentially lunches the next day. Be sure to add in fresh items to make breakfasts and prepare snacks. Organic or local fresh farm raised items are preferred.

Double check your stock pantry list to make sure you have the essentials. If you have made your meat rub, taco seasoning and breading, the "aisle" ingredients will be minimal. Spices can be purchased in larger quantities online.

MEATS

Unless otherwise specified, the recommended serving size will depend on the number of portions. The recommended amount of meat/fish per serving is 1/2 pound.

- [ ] whole chicken or 4 chicken breasts (for white chicken chili)
- [ ] 1-2 pounds of grass-fed ground beef (for tomato sauce; if you have frozen sauce from week 1, you may omit this ingredient)
- [ ] 2-3 pounds of grass-fed beef (for burgers)
- [ ] white fish or salmon-avoid tilapia (for spiced dry rubbed steak)

REFRIGERATED SECTION

- [ ] eggs (1 dozen NEEDED for egg parmesan, purchase additional as needed for breakfast)
- [ ] nut milk (unsweetened)
- [ ] coconut yogurt (plain/unsweetened; no more than 1-2 grams of sugar)
- [ ] Pecorino Romano cheese (check local wholesale clubs for value; for egg parmesan)

AISLE

- [ ] coconut and/or olive oil
- [ ] Dijon mustard
- [ ] pickles (avoid artificial dyes)
- [ ] 4 cans of white beans
- [ ] cumin
- [ ] oregano
- [ ] dried Italian spices
- [ ] coconut flour**
- [ ] almond flour**
- [ ] sunflower seeds**
- [ ] lentils (dried, spouted or 2 cans)
- [ ] slivered almonds (for buttery green beans)
- [ ] apple cider vinegar

**Omit these ingredients if breading is already prepped

Depending on which chicken or fish recipe you have chosen for this week, add ingredients to your grocery list.

WEEK THREE GROCERIES

PRODUCE

- ☐ 1 butternut squash (pre-cut and frozen available, for vegetable medley)
- ☐ 1 bunch of asparagus (for vegetable medley)
- ☐ 1 red onion (for vegetable medley)
- ☐ 1 red bell pepper (for vegetable medley)
- ☐ 1 head cauliflower (for vegetable medley)
- ☐ 1 zucchini (for vegetable medley)
- ☐ 1 celery (for soup)
- ☐ 4-6 boxes of tomatoes/fresh tomatoes (for sauce)
- ☐ jalapeños (optional for white bean chili)
- ☐ 1 bunch of chard (for tomato sauce)
- ☐ avocados (enjoy in moderation)
- ☐ berries (enjoy in moderation)
- ☐ grapefruit (enjoy in moderation)
- ☐ sweet potatoes (optional to add to chicken or fish)
- ☐ 1 small bag of carrots (fresh, pre-cut or frozen for lentil soup)
- ☐ 6 fresh onions or 3 bags of frozen onions
- ☐ 1 bunch of collard greens (fresh or frozen for white chicken chili)
- ☐ 2 bunches of cilantro (for white chicken chili and burgers)
- ☐ basil and parsley (for tomato sauce)
- ☐ garlic (fresh, jarred or frozen)
- ☐ lemon juice (omit if not making marinade for chicken)
- ☐ 1 spaghetti squash (vegetable noodles can be substituted; base for egg parmesan)
- ☐ green beans (fresh or frozen; to substitute for fries with burger)
- ☐ lettuce for salad (spinach, romaine, mixed greens, arugula, etc.)
- ☐ 1 cucumber (for cucumber and tomato salad)
- ☐ 1 package of grape tomatoes (for cucumber and tomato salad)

This list includes items you will need for dinners and most lunches. Be sure to add items you will need for breakfasts and other members of your household.

WEEK FOUR

CARBOHYDRATES

Carbohydrates are a major macronutrient and one of the body's primary sources of energy. The debate about whether to eat carbs seems to be a constant diet fad. There are two different types of carbohydrates, simple and complex, and the way your body process simple is very different than complex.

SIMPLE CARBOHYDRATES

Simple carbohydrates are sugar. Your body breaks them down almost instantly, affecting your blood sugar in an often drastic way. These include cereal, white bread, baked goods and most packaged snacks. Fruit juice concentrate and soda are also frequent offenders.

COMPLEX CARBOHYDRATES

Complex carbohydrates pack in more nutrients than simple carbs because they are higher in fiber and they digest more slowly. They also help to minimize blood sugar spikes. The two classifications of complex carbohydrates are fiber and starch. The main sources of fiber are fruits, vegetables, nuts and beans. The more starchy types of complex carbs include corn, oats, potatoes and rice.

RESISTANT CARBOHYDRATES

Resistant starches are starches that resist digestion in the small intestine and pass through to the large intestine. In doing this, they are much more slowly metabolized and often times act similarly to fiber minimizing these foods impact on blood sugar. The starch in seeds and legumes resists digestion because the starch is bound to the cell walls. The resistant starch feeds the good bacteria in the gut lining.

A good way to implement resistant starch in lifelong eating would be to enjoy a rice pasta for dinner, refrigerat it overnight and then enjoy cold the next day. Cold potato salad is also a great way to use this tip. The starch must be cooled completely and refrigerated for 6 to 8 hours in order to make it resistant. It can be left at room temperature or heated up to 100°. If it is heated beyond that, the starch is no longer resistant. Raw potatoes and bananas that aren't fully ripe also have an indigestible starch. Potatoes and rice that are cooked, then cooled (6-8 hours) turn a traditional starch into a resistant starch.

PHASE THREE

WEEK 4
CARBOHYDRATES

CARBOHYDRATES ARE A MAJOR MACRONUTRIENT AND ONE OF THE BODY'S PRIMARY SOURCES OF ENERGY. THERE ARE TWO DIFFERENT TYPES OF CARBOHYDRATES: **SIMPLE AND COMPLEX** AND THE WAY YOUR BODY PROCESSES BOTH **IS VERY DIFFERENT**

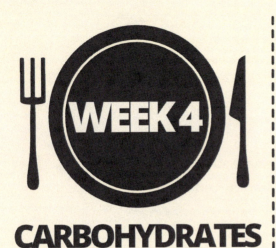

SIMPLE

SIMPLE CARBOHYDRATES ARE **SUGAR**

YOUR BODY BREAKS THEM DOWN **ALMOST INSTANTLY** AFFECTING YOUR BLOOD SUGAR IN **OFTEN DRASTIC WAYS**

THESE INCLUDE CEREAL, WHITE BREAD, BAKED GOODS, AND MOST PACKAGED SNACKS

FRUIT JUICE CONCENTRATE AND **SODA** ARE ALSO FREQUENT OFFENDERS

COMPLEX

PACK **MORE NUTRIENTS** BECAUSE THEY ARE **HIGHER IN FIBER** AND THEY **DIGEST MORE SLOWLY**

MINIMIZE BLOOD SUGAR SPIKES

THE TWO CLASSIFICATIONS: **FIBER** AND **STARCH**

THE MAIN SOURCES OF FIBER ARE **FRUITS, VEGETABLES, NUTS AND BEANS**

THE MORE STARCHY TYPES OF COMPLEX CARBS INCLUDE **CORN, OATS, POTATOES, AND RICE**

RESISTANT STARCH

STARCHES THAT RESIST DIGESTION IN THE SMALL INTESTINE AND PASS THROUGH TO THE LARGE INTESTINE

MUCH MORE SLOWLY METABOLIZED AND OFTEN TIMES ACT SIMILARLY TO FIBER, MINIMIZING THESE FOODS IMPACT ON BLOOD SUGARS. THE STARCH IN SEEDS AND LEGUMES RESIST DIGESTION DUE TO THE FACT THAT THE STARCH IS BOUND TO THE CELL WALLS

RAW POTATOES AND BANANAS THAT AREN'T FULLY RIPE ALSO HAVE AN INDIGESTIBLE STARCH. POTATOES AND RICE THAT ARE COOKED THEN COOLED (6-8 HOURS) TURN A TRADITIONAL STARCH INTO A RESISTANT STARCH.

LOAD UP! WEEK FOUR

Please continue to load up on the same ingredients that were in Weeks 1-3. Use moderation in continuing to introduce new items.

MEATS
(Pasture raised or organic is best)
beef, bison, lamb

POULTRY
(Pasture raised or organic is best)
chicken, duck, turkey, cornish game hens

FISH
(Wild caught is best)
Cod, Grouper, Mahi Mahi, Snapper, Tuna, Sole Orange Roughy, Haddock, Salmon, Trout

EGGS
(Pasture raised hens are best)
chicken eggs, duck eggs

DAIRY
goats or sheep milk products, raw or organic cream (for coffee), raw or organic milk (in small amounts)

FATS & OILS
avocado, butter, coconut oil, olive oil, organic ghee

VEGETABLES
(organic, fresh or frozen) ALL vegetables, white potatoes, corn (non GMO), sweet potatoes (keep to fist sized portions)

SWEETENERS
coconut sugar, whole cane sugar (unprocessed), honey, maple syrup, stevia

BEANS & LEGUMES
black beans, navy beans, white beans, kidney beans, garbanzo beans

NUTS & SEEDS
(unprocessed/raw)
almonds, cashews, chia, coconut, flaxseed, hazelnut, hempseed, macadamia, pecans, pumpkin, sunflower, walnuts, nuts/seed butters

SPICES
(suggested, but not limited to)
basil, Celtic sea salt, cumin, cinnamon, cracked pepper, ginger, Himalayan salt, rosemary, thyme, turmeric, paprika, Italian seasoning, onion, garlic, vanilla, anything that doesn't contain sugar

FRUITS
ALL fruits, limit those high in fructose

BEVERAGES
an occasional alcoholic beverage is permitted (avoiding is best)

HERBS
(organic, fresh, or frozen) basil, parsley, dill, oregano, cilantro, sage rosemary, mint

STEER CLEAR! WEEK FOUR

MEATS
pork

FISH
shellfish

EGGS
imitation eggs, Egg Beaters

DAIRY
soy milk (GMO)

FATS & OILS
canola oil (GMO), corn oil, lard, safflower oil, margarine, soybean oil, cottonseed oil, hydrogenated or partially hydrogenated oils

BEANS & LEGUMES
soy beans, tofu

NUTS & SEEDS
dry, roasted in oil, honey roasted

CONDIMENTS/SPICES
any that contain added sugar (read the label)

FRUITS
See page 37 for guide

BEVERAGES
alcoholic (limited), ABSOLUTELY NO soda

GRAINS
breads, pastas, rice, cereal, pastries, baked goods (anything with flour)

SWEETENERS
sugar, high fructose corn syrup, sugar alcohol, xylitol, sorbitol, all artificial sweeteners

WEEK FOUR MEALS

BREAKFAST

These are suggested breakfast items. Breakfast may be substituted with a shake balanced in proteins, fats and carbs.

EGGS: scrambled, boiled, fried, omelette (add herbs, onions, tomatoes, greens and/or avocado)

FRITTATA MUFFIN

GRAINLESS GRANOLA (1/4-1/3 cup)

GRAINLESS WAFFLES

SHAKE can be used as a meal replacement

CHIA PUDDING (1/4-1/2 cup)

DINNER

You may eat the meals in the order you choose.

PIZZA with salad

PASTA PRIMAVERA, SWEET POTATO NOODLES and salad

CHICKEN FINGERS with **RAW VEGGIES** and Ceasar salad

ROAST BEEF & CAULIFLOWER MASH with salad

BUTTERNUT SQUASH SOUP with salad

PURPOSEFUL LEFTOVERS

DINE OUT to challenge yourself to make great choices.

LUNCH

Lunches should be purposeful leftovers from dinner the night before. Leftovers can be accompanied by :

SOUP

RAW VEGETABLES

BOILED EGG

OLIVES (3-5)

GOAT OR SHEEP MILK CHEESE small amount

FRESH MIXED GREENS topped with protein

SNACKS

These are approved snacks that are optional. Be mindful to combine a protein, a fat and a carbohydrate with snack options.

- **CARSON'S CRACKERS**
- **HARD BOILED EGGS**
- **SICILIAN SPICED OLIVES**
- **PECORINO ROMANO CHEESE**
- **NUTS/NUT BUTTER**
- **UNSALTED SEEDS**
- **PROTEIN SHAKE WITH COCONUT MILK**
- **GRANOLA/POWER BALLS**
- **AVOCADO/WHOLE FRUIT/ VEGGIES**

Read and understand your labels. Be mindful of unhealthy salt & oils.

Portions

complex carbs   protein   healthy fat   snack

WEEK FOUR GROCERIES

This list includes items you will use for dinner and potentially lunches the next day. Be sure to add in fresh items to make breakfasts and prepare snacks. Organic or local fresh farm raised items are preferred.

Double check your stock pantry list to make sure you have the essentials. If you have made your meat rub, taco seasoning and breading, the "aisle" ingredients will be minimal. Spices can be purchased in larger quantities online.

MEATS

Unless otherwise specified, the recommended serving size will depend on the number of portions. The recommended amount of meat/fish per serving is 1/2 pound.

- [ ] 3 pounds chicken breasts/tenders
- [ ] 3-4 pounds beef roast
- [ ] pizza topping of your choice (read ingredients)

REFRIGERATED SECTION

- [ ] eggs
- [ ] Pecorino Romano cheese
- [ ] 3-4 ounces fresh mozarella (per pizza)
- [ ] sour cream/whipping cream (optional)
- [ ] coconut yogurt

AISLE

- [ ] coconut and/or olive oil
- [ ] pesto sauce with olive oil (for pizza crust)
- [ ] dried Italian spices
- [ ] garlic powder*
- [ ] flax seed*
- [ ] sesame seed*
- [ ] hemp seeds*
- [ ] paprika*
- [ ] coconut sugar*
- [ ] Himalayan salt
- [ ] 1 cup coconut flour**
- [ ] 1 cup almond flour**
- [ ] sunflower seeds**
- [ ] red wine
- [ ] beef broth
- [ ] 1-2 jars of tomato puree

*Omit these ingredients if dry rub is already prepped

**Omit these ingredients if breading is already prepped

WEEK FOUR GROCERIES

PRODUCE

- [ ] 2 butternut squash (pre-cut for soup)
- [ ] 3-4 apples (for soup)
- [ ] 1 small bag of carrots (frozen, pre-cut for soup)
- [ ] 2 heads of cauliflower (1 for mash, 1 for pasta primavera)
- [ ] 2-3 bags pre-chopped cauli-bits (for pizza crust)
- [ ] 1 bunch of asparagus (for pasta primavera)
- [ ] 2-3 red bell peppers (for pasta primavera and pizza topping)
- [ ] 2 zucchini (for pasta primavera and pizza topping)
- [ ] 1 purple onion (for pasta primavera)
- [ ] 4 white onions (for roast)
- [ ] 1-2 bags of frozen onions (for soup)
- [ ] 8 ounces of sliced mushrooms (optional, for pizza)
- [ ] 2-3 cups fresh spinach (for pizza topping)
- [ ] fresh basil
- [ ] fresh parsley
- [ ] 2-3 heads of garlic (fresh, frozen, or jarred)
- [ ] lettuce for salad (Romaine, Kale, etc.)
- [ ] sweet potatoes, zucchini or squash (to cut into noodles)
- [ ] berries (enjoy in moderation)
- [ ] grapefruits (enjoy in moderation)
- [ ] greens (for salads)
- [ ] fresh herbs

This list includes items you will need for dinners and most lunches. Be sure to add items you will need for breakfasts and other members of your household.

METABOLICALLY SPEAKING

Humans are the only species that seek advice and experiment with different diets. In the wild, there are carnivores, omnivores and herbivores that innately feast on meat, meat and plants, and plants only, respectively. We as humans are innately wired differently within our species. Some of us metabolize more like a carnivore (tiger) requiring more protein and fat than others. Some of us metabolize like an omnivore (bear) and require a more balanced ratio of macro nutrients. Some of us resemble herbivores (deer) requiring more carbohydrates as others.

So what am I? A tiger? A bear? Or a deer?

An estimated 65% of us are wired more like the omnivorous bear. 10% of us are innately wired like the carnivorous tiger leaving 25% of us to be wired like the herbivorous deer, grazing throughout their days.

How do I find out what I am and how I should be eating for my metabolism?

By resetting your body and eating clean, you have already reclaimed your taste buds. By taking steps like eliminating sugar, cutting cravings and making better choices, you have put yourself in a parasympathetic state and are far more in touch with your own innate metabolism. I suggest going straight to the source of the metabolic diet research. William Walcott and Trish Fahey authored a book called "The Metabolic Typing Diet." It helps you to free yourself from food cravings, achieve your ideal weight, enjoy high energy and robust health, all the while preventing and reversing disease. This book is a wealth of information on this topic. There is also a genetic marker called "APO E" that can be detected in a blood test. This genetic marker determines which type you are.

In a nut shell, APO E 2's metabolize more like carnivorous tigers and are referred to as the protein type.
APO E3's are more like the omnivorous bear and are referred to as the mixed type.
APOE 4's are wired like the herbivorous deer and are referred to as carb types.

All three types of people require all three macro nutrients—proteins, fats and carbohydrates. The difference is, different types of people require different ratios of those macro nutrients. A guideline is shown below.

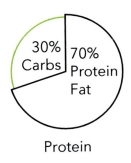

Protein

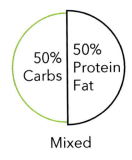

Mixed

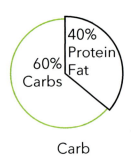

Carb

IF YOU ARE A MIXED TYPE...

Your metabolism is as unique as your finger print. You are not exactly like anyone else! However, there are a few things you may have in common with other protein types: a moderate appetite, no strong cravings for sugars or sweets, and if you stick to your plate, you will rarely have a weight problem. The mixed type diet is the most liberal. It is a mix of the protein type and the carb type diets. While the other two have some "forbidden foods," you can eat everything! Your challenge is to work on finding your personal code. Which of these foods do you thrive on?

SIMPLE RULES TO LIVE BY FOR THE MIXED TYPE

- Be sure to eat protein at every meal.
- Each day mix your high purine and low purine proteins.
- Snack as needed with balance (Protein, Carbohydrate, Fat).
- Dairy products need to be removed and reintroduced
- Choose both starchy/non-starchy carbohydrates and combine.
- Use grains (whole/ancient) in moderation: Limit bread.
- Use juices cautiously: more vegetable juice with limited fruit juices.
- Regulate your blood sugar and monitor with a glucose meter.

INTRODUCING NEW FOODS

To find out what foods you do best on, start with eliminating all grains (corn, wheat, rice, etc), all sugar (refined, natural and especially artificial) and dairy (limited goat or sheep milk permitted) for a period of 2 weeks. When you introduce foods back into the diet, follow these rules and journal how you feel. This will determine if you should add them back in or avoid them.

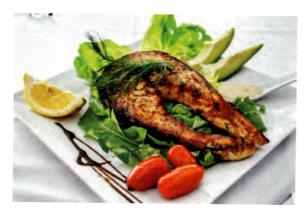

Introduce one food item at a time and pay attention to how it makes you feel for the next 24-48 hours.

Abstain 24-48 hours before introducing another food item. If you put back dairy and potatoes, then don't feel well, you want to know which the culprit is!

Introduce them in the following order: Vegetable (starchy), then sweet/white potatoes, then a whole grain bread (sprouted grain recommended) and journal, journal, journal!

MIXED FOOD "PYRAMID"

PRIMARY FOODS 🟨 🟦 🟥

LOW GLYCEMIC VEGETABLES

Lettuce(s), Arugula, Beet Greens, Broccoli Raabe, Spring Mix, Seaweeds, Endive, Brussels Sprouts, Cabbage, Bok Choy, Radicchio, Cucumber, Horseradish, Radish, Leek, Bell Pepper, Broccoli, Cilantro, Parsley, Sprouts, Egg Plant, Fennel, Ginger Root, Onion, Scallion, Shallot, Garlic, Tomato, Chard, Kale, Mustard Greens, Turnip Greens, Collard Greens, Dandelion Greens, Celery, Mushrooms, Spinach, Asparagus, Cauliflower, String Beans

MEAT, FISH & FOWL

Chicken Breast*, Cornish Hen*, Turkey Breast*, Cod*, Flounder*, Grouper*, Haddock*, Halibut*, Mahi Mahi*, Eggs (Whole)*, Cheese*, Cottage Cheese*, Perch*, Red Snapper*, Sole*, Trout*, Tuna*, White Sea Bass*

Heart**, Kidney, Pate**, Organ Meats**, Anchovy**, Herring**, Sardine**, Arctic Char**, Tuna**, Dark (Ahi)**, Mussel**, Clam**, Crab**, Crawfish**, Lobster**, Oyster**, Scallop**, Shrimp**, Snail**, Beef**, Liver**, Beef**, Lamb**, Goat**, Buffalo**, Veal**, Venison**, Wild Game**, Chicken (Dark)**, Turkey (Dark)**, Chicken Liver**, Pheasant**, Ostrich**, Goose**, Duck**, Quail**, Pork Chop**, Bacon**, Ham**, Spare Rib**, Caviare**, Mackerel**, Octopus**, Salmon**, Squid**

Limit pork & shellfish consumption for optimal health
Low Purine Fish & Fowl
***High Purine Meat, Fish & Fowl*

HIGH FAT SEEDS & NUTS

Coconut, Olives, Butter, Cream, Ghee, Coconut Oil, Olive Oil, Avocado, Milk, Yogurt, Almond, Cashew, Filbert/Hazel, Flax Seed, Macadamia, Peanut, Pecan, Pine Nuts, Pistachio, Pumpkin, Sesame, Sunflower, Walnut

HIGH GLYCEMIC VEGETABLES, FRUITS & GRAINS

Artichoke, Beet, Carrot, Jicama, Okra, Peas, Pumpkin, Rutabaga, Spaghetti Squash, Beans (dry), Lentils, Peas (dry), Banana, Cantaloupe, Grapefruit, Kiwi, Lemon, Lime, Mango, Orange, Papaya, Pineapple, Pomegranate, Tangerine, Watermelon, Cranberries, Lemon, Lime, Pomegranate, Apple, Apricot, Blackberry, Blueberry, Cherries, Figs, Grapes, Nectarines, Peach, Pear, Persimmon, Raspberry, Strawberry, Plum, All Other Berries, All Other Melons, Corn (on the cob), Amaranth, Brown Rice, Buckwheat, Millet, Oat, Quinoa, Wild Rice, Chestnut, Summer Squash, Turnip, Yellow Squash, Zucchini, Parsnip, Potato, Jerusalem Artichoke, Sweet Potato, Winter Squash, Yam

SECONDARY FOODS 🟩

IF YOU ARE A PROTEIN TYPE...

Your metabolism is as unique as your finger print. You are not exactly like anyone else! However, there are a few things you may have in common with other protein types: a strong appetite, a preference for salty, fatty foods, and issues with fatigue, anxiety or nervousness. By eating higher amounts of protein and fat in comparison to carbohydrates, you will better meet your needs. As a protein type, your body converts carbohydrates into energy too quickly. Heavier foods rich in protein and fat slow down the rate of oxidation.

SIMPLE RULES TO LIVE BY FOR THE PROTEIN TYPE

- Eat protein every meal (high purine proteins preferred).
- Do not eat carbohydrates alone. For example, don't eat an apple alone, eat it with nut butter.
- Beware of bread. Stick to whole grains.
- Juicing is limited, avoid fruit juice when possible.
- Freely use HEALTHY fats and oils.
- It is recommended that you eat your protein first, then your carbohydrates.

INTRODUCING NEW FOODS

To find out what foods you do best on, start with eliminating all grains (corn, wheat, rice, etc), all sugar (refined, natural and especially artificial) and dairy (limited goat or sheep milk permitted) for a period of 2 weeks. When you introduce foods back into the diet, follow these rules and journal how you feel. This will determine if you should add them back in or avoid them.

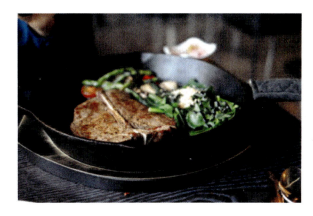

Introduce one food item at a time and pay attention to how it makes you feel for the next 24-48 hours.

Abstain 24-48 hours before introducing another food item. If you put back dairy and potatoes, then don't feel well, you want to know which the culprit is!

Introduce them in the following order: Vegetable (starchy), then sweet/white potatoes, then a whole grain bread (sprouted grain recommended) and journal, journal, journal!

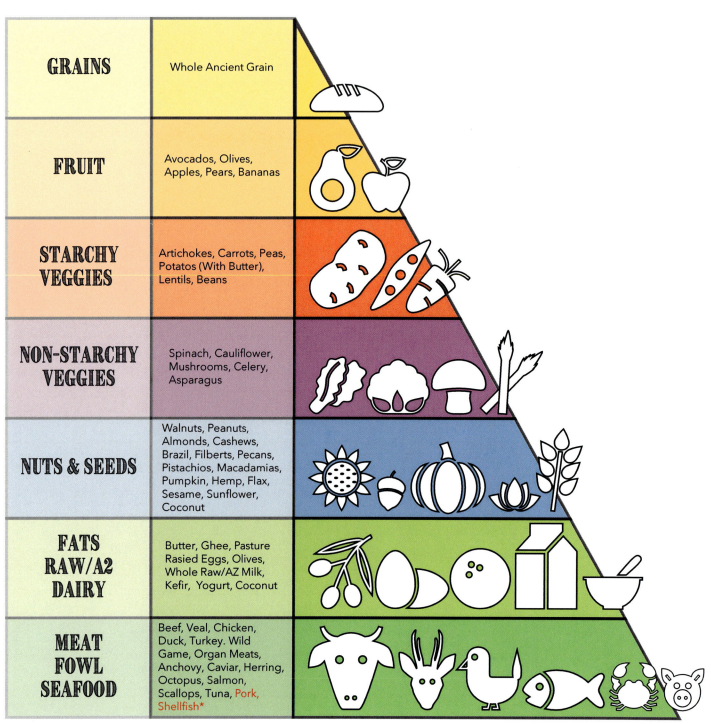

IF YOU ARE A CARB TYPE...

Your metabolism is as unique as your finger print. You are not exactly like anyone else! However, there are a few things you may have in common with other protein types: a relatively weak appetite, a high tolerance for sweets, a lean body type (at least most start that way), tendency towards a Type A personality and caffeine dependency. Your needs as a carbohydrate type are comprised of smaller amount of proteins and fats in comparison to carbohydrates. The proteins suggested for you are lower purine (or lighter fare). You can tolerate a wide and abundant variety of vegetables and fruits. Grains are also permissible for your type. Although you tolerate sugar and sweets, be careful not to overdo it as it leads to health issues and blood sugar related illness. You tend to slowly metabolize your foods which is why large amounts of protein and fat are not recommended. Choose low protein and foods with naturally occurring lower fat choices, but not "fat-free" or "low-fat" products.

SIMPLE RULES TO LIVE BY FOR THE CARB TYPE

- Choose lower fat and low purine proteins over others
- Eat protein with most but not all meals.
- Choose lower fat dairy like yogurts and cottage cheese.
- Most dairy is not ideal.
- Balance your carb intake between starchy and non starchy.
- Enjoy vegetable juices and fruit juices
- Minimize fats and oils.
- DO NOT cut out fat. It's necessary for proper cell functions.
- Eat limited nuts and seeds.
- Snack as needed.
- Enjoy your bread (ancient whole grains and sprouted grain is best.

INTRODUCING NEW FOODS

To find out what foods you do best on, start with eliminating all grains (corn, wheat, rice, etc), all sugar (refined, natural and especially artificial) and dairy (limited goat or sheep milk permitted) for a period of 2 weeks. When you introduce foods back into the diet, follow these rules and journal how you feel. This will determine if you should add them back in or avoid them.

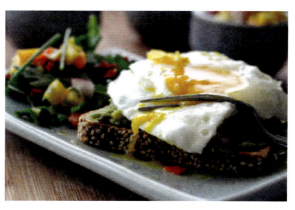

Introduce one food item at a time and pay attention to how it makes you feel for the next 24-48 hours.

Abstain 24-48 hours before introducing another food item. If you put back dairy and potatoes, then don't feel well, you want to know which the culprit is!

Introduce them in the following order: Vegetable (starchy), then sweet/white potatoes, then a whole grain bread (sprouted grain recommended) and journal, journal, journal!

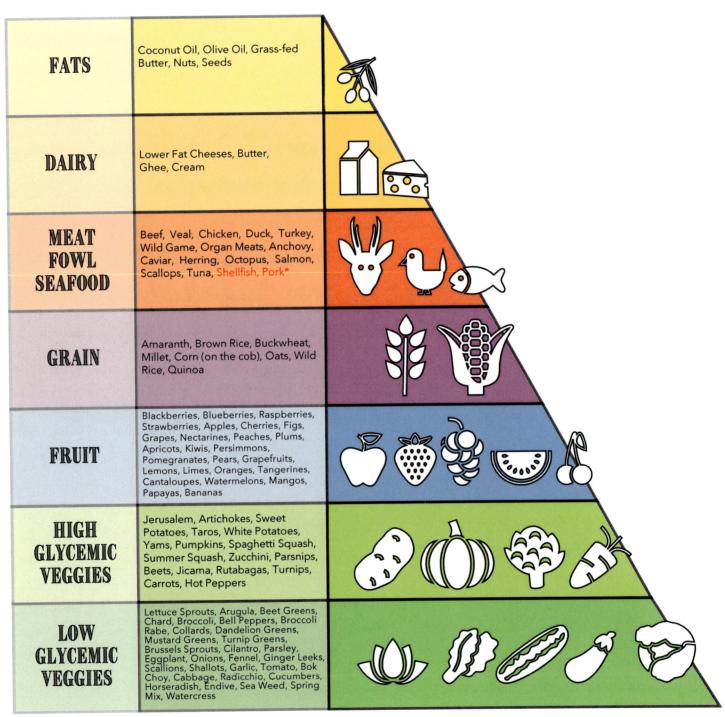

WEEK FIVE MEALS

BREAKFAST

These are suggested breakfast items. Breakfast may be substituted with a shake, balanced in proteins, fats, and carbs.

EGGS: scrambled, boiled, fried, omelette (add herbs, onions, tomatoes, greens and/or avocado)

FRITTATA MUFFIN

GRAINLESS GRANOLA (1/4-1/3 cup)

CHIA PUDDING (1/4-1/2 cup)

DINNER

You may eat the meals in the order you choose.

LEMON CHICKEN with Ceaser salad

VEGETABLE SPAGHETTI & BOLOGNESE SAUCE

PAPA'S CHICKEN SOUP with salad

5 HOUR STEW with salad (make the day before)

SESAME CRUSTED SALMON with veggie medley

PURPOSEFUL LEFTOVERS

DINE OUT to challenge yourself to make great choices.

LUNCH

Lunches should be purposeful leftovers from dinner the night before. Leftovers can be accompanied by :

SOUP

RAW OR COOKED VEGETABLES

BOILED EGG

OLIVES (3-5)

FRESH MIXED GREENS (1/4-1/2 cup)

SNACKS

These are approved snacks that are optional. Be mindful to combine a protein, a fat and a carbohydrate with snack options.

- CARSON'S CRACKERS
- HARD BOILED EGGS
- SICILIAN SPICED OLIVES
- PECORINO ROMANO CHEESE
- NUTS/NUT BUTTER
- UNSALTED SEEDS
- PROTEIN SHAKE WITH COCONUT MILK
- GRANOLA/POWER BALLS
- AVOCADO/WHOLE FRUIT/ VEGGIES

Read and understand your labels. Be mindful of unhealthy salt & oils.

Portions:

 complex carbs

 protein

 healthy fat

 snack

PHASE FOUR

WEEK FIVE GROCERIES

This list includes items you will use for dinner and potentially lunches the next day. Be sure to add in fresh items to make breakfasts and prepare snacks. Organic or local fresh farm raised items are preferred.

Double check your stock pantry list to make sure you have the essentials.

MEATS

Unless otherwise specifiied, the recommended serving size will depend on the number of portions. The recommended amount of meat/fish per serving is 1/2 pound.

- ☐ whole chicken (for soup)
- ☐ 3-4 pounds of steak/stewing beef (for stew)
- ☐ 1-2 pounds of ground meat (for meat sauce)
- ☐ wild caught salmon filet (chicken substitute)
- ☐ chicken breasts (for marinated chicken or Ceasar salad)

AISLE

- ☐ tobasco
- ☐ worcestershire
- ☐ Dijon mustard
- ☐ red wine vinegar
- ☐ red wine
- ☐ 5-24 oz of tomatoes (not canned)
- ☐ coconut/olive oil
- ☐ dried Italian spices
- ☐ Himalayan salt
- ☐ beef broth
- ☐ anchovy paste (optional)

REFRIGERATED SECTION

- ☐ 1-2 dozen eggs
- ☐ coconut/almond milk (unsweetened)
- ☐ Pecorino Romano Cheese (whole or grated)

PRODUCE

- ☐ 2 bags of carrots (fresh or frozen)
- ☐ onions (4-6 fresh or 3 bags frozen)
- ☐ 2 bunches of celery (pre-chopped optional)
- ☐ red bell pepper (for medley)
- ☐ butternut squash (1 fresh or 2 bags frozen)
- ☐ turnip greens (fresh or frozen)
- ☐ spaghetti squash OR zucchini (1 per person)
- ☐ bunch asparagus (for medley)
- ☐ zucchini (for medley)
- ☐ head caulifower (pre-cut for medley)
- ☐ 3-4 lemons or bottled lemon juice
- ☐ 1 package of fresh dill
- ☐ basil (fresh or frozen)
- ☐ 1 bunch of fresh parsley (for soup)
- ☐ 1 bunch of Swiss chard (for Bolognese)

This list includes items you will need for dinners and most lunches. Be sure to add items you will need for breakfasts and other members of your household.

GOAL SETTING

What is a goal? A goal is where you want to be, something you would like to achieve. Developing longterm goals and working backwards to create a plan brings organization and a great deal of clarity to the actions and decisions that you need to make now.

Goals should be SMART - Specific, Measurable, Attainable, Realistic and Timely

Specific: simple, detailed, particular, focused, easy to understand.
Measurable: quantifiable, how will you know if you achieved it?
Attainable: something that does not depend on others to achieve. You alone are responsible for it.
Realistic: something that is not too hard or too easy, but is in reach and requires some growth and effort.
Timely: give yourself an exact deadline!

Use this template to write down your goals, whether they're physical, emotional, spiritual, or professional. Write them down!

GOALS

Long Term

Short Term

Action Steps Required

1.

2.

3.

Who Will Be Involved?	What Will Be Required?
When Will You Work on It?	How Will You know?

WEEK SIX MEALS

BREAKFAST

These are suggested breakfast items. Breakfast may be substituted with a shake, balanced in proteins, fats and carbs.

EGGS: scrambled, boiled, fried, omelette (add herbs, onions, tomatoes, greens and/or avocado)

FRITTATA MUFFIN

GRAINLESS GRANOLA (1/4-1/3 cup)

CHIA PUDDING (1/4-1/2 cup)

DINNER

You may eat the meals in the order you choose.

TACO SALAD (beef OR chicken) with cilantro lime dressing

PAPA'S MINESTRONE with salad

HERB ROASTED CHICKEN with garden salad (freeze carcass for week eight)

ALMOND CRUSTED FISH with vegetable medley

DRY RUBBED STEAK & CAULIFLOWER MASH with spinach

PURPOSEFUL LEFTOVERS

DINE OUT to challenge yourself to make great choices.

LUNCH

Lunches should be purposeful leftovers from dinner the night before. Leftovers can be accompanied by :

SOUP

RAW OR COOKED VEGETABLES

BOILED EGG

OLIVES (3-5)

FRESH MIXED GREENS topped with protein

SNACKS

These are approved snacks that are optional. Use as recommended by your doctor. Be mindful to combine a protein, a fat and a carbohydrate with snack options.

- CARSON'S CRACKERS
- HARD BOILED EGGS
- SICILIAN SPICED OLIVES
- PECORINO ROMANO CHEESE
- NUTS/NUT BUTTER
- UNSALTED SEEDS
- PROTEIN SHAKE WITH COCONUT MILK
- GRANOLA/POWER BALLS
- AVOCADO/WHOLE FRUIT/ VEGGIES

Read and understand your labels. Be mindful of unhealthy salt & oils.

Portions

complex carbs | protein | healthy fat | snack

PHASE FOUR

WEEK SIX GROCERIES

This list includes items you will use for dinner and potentially lunches the next day. Be sure to add in fresh items to make breakfasts and prepare snacks. Organic or local fresh farm raised items are preferred.

Double check your stock pantry list to make sure you have the essentials. If you have made your meat rub, taco seasoning and breading, the "aisle" ingredients will be minimal. Spices can be purchased in larger quantities online.

MEATS

Unless otherwise specified, the recommended serving size will depend on the number of portions. The recommended amount of meat/fish per serving is 1/2 pound.

- ☐ 1 whole chicken (for herb roasted chicken)
- ☐ 2 pounds of ground beef or chicken (taco salad)
- ☐ 2-3 pounds of grass-fed ground beef (omit if you have leftover meatballs)
- ☐ white fish (chicken may be substituted)
- ☐ grass fed-steaks (for spiced dry rubbed steak)

REFRIGERATED SECTION

- ☐ eggs for breakfast & hard boiled (for snacks/taco salad)
- ☐ coconut milk (unsweetened)
- ☐ coconut yogurt (plain/unsweetened; no more than 1-2 grams of sugar)
- ☐ Pecorino Romano cheese 3 cups (check local wholesale clubs for value; for breading and as a soup topper)

AISLE

- ☐ coconut and/or olive oil
- ☐ dried Italian herbs
- ☐ Himalayan salt
- ☐ cumin
- ☐ granulated garlic
- ☐ organic soy sauce (Tamari or Braggs liquid amino)
- ☐ sesame seeds
- ☐ hemp seeds/hearts
- ☐ paprika
- ☐ chili powder
- ☐ slivered almonds
- ☐ dried onion
- ☐ Dijon mustard
- ☐ apple cider vinegar
- ☐ balsamic vinegar
- ☐ turmeric
- ☐ almond flour
- ☐ coconut flour
- ☐ 2 cups red wine (for cooking)
- ☐ organic coffee grounds (steak dry rub optional)

This list includes items you will need for dinners and most lunches. Be sure to add items you will need for breakfasts and other members of your household.

WEEK SIX GROCERIES

PRODUCE

- ☐ carrots (1 fresh for chicken, 1 frozen for soup)
- ☐ 1 bag of frozen peas (for minestrone soup; frozen peas and carrots are available together)
- ☐ onions (3-4 fresh or 2 bags of pre-cut frozen for soup and taco salad)
- ☐ 1 bunch fresh cilantro (taco salad dressing)
- ☐ 1 head of iceberg lettuce (taco salad)
- ☐ 1 purple onion (available pre-chopped)
- ☐ 1 bunch of celery (pre-chopped optional) (for soup)
- ☐ collard greens 1 bunch fresh or 1 bag frozen (for minestrone)
- ☐ 1-2 red bell peppers (for vegetable medley and taco salad)
- ☐ 1 jalapeño pepper (for salad dressing—omit if you do not like spicy)
- ☐ butternut squash (purchase pre-chopped or frozen) (for vegetable medley)
- ☐ 2 bunches of asparagus (for vegetable medley and steak dinner)
- ☐ 1 zucchini (for vegetable medley)
- ☐ cauliflower (for vegetable medley; pre-cut fresh)
- ☐ 1 bag frozen cauliflower (for cauliflower mash)
- ☐ 1-2 bags of spinach (fresh or frozen)
- ☐ 2-3 limes or bottled lime juice and 6 lemons
- ☐ basil fresh or frozen cubes (for tomato sauce)
- ☐ fresh parsley, chives, sage, thyme, rosemary (for herb roasted chicken)
- ☐ organic soy sauce/tamari, dijon mustard, 2 cups of lemon juice (for herb roasted chicken)
- ☐ 2-3 heads of fresh garlic, jarred or frozen
- ☐ lettuce for salads (romaine, iceberg, spinach, kale, arugula, mixed greens)
- ☐ 1 cucumber (taco salad)
- ☐ 2-3 avocados (taco salad/taco salad dressing)
- ☐ 2 pounds of fresh tomatoes or jarred/boxed diced (for minestrone)
- ☐ 1 package of grape tomatoes (for taco salad)
- ☐ salad toppers (fresh veggies you prefer)
- ☐ nuts and seeds (pumpkin seeds top the taco salad for crunch)

WEEK SEVEN MEALS

BREAKFAST

These are suggested breakfast items. Breakfast may be substituted with a shake, balanced in proteins, fats and carbs.

EGGS: scrambled, boiled, fried, omelette (add herbs, onions, tomatoes, greens and/or avocado)

FRITTATA MUFFIN

GRAINLESS GRANOLA (1/4-1/3 cup)

SHAKE can be used as a meal replacement

CHIA PUDDING (1/4-1/2 cup)

EGGS FOR A CROWD

DINNER

You may eat the meals in the order you choose.

LENTIL SOUP with salad (add meat optional)

BEEF BURGERS WITH BUTTERY GREEN BEANS and salad

CHICKEN/FISH recipe of your choice and **VEGETABLE MEDLEY** with salad

EGGPLANT PARMIGIANA & VEGETABLE PASTA with salad

WHITE BEAN CHICKEN CHILI with salad

PURPOSEFUL LEFTOVERS

DINE OUT to challenge yourself to make great choices.

LUNCH

Lunches should be purposeful leftovers from dinner the night before. Leftovers can be accompanied by :

SOUP

RAW OR COOKED VEGETABLES

BOILED EGG

OLIVES (3-5)

GOAT OR SHEEP MILK CHEESE small amount

FRESH MIXED GREENS topped with protein

SNACKS

These are approved snacks that are optional. Be mindful to combine a protein, a fat and a carbohydrate with snack options.

- CARSON'S CRACKERS
- HARD BOILED EGGS
- SICILIAN SPICED OLIVES
- PECORINO ROMANO CHEESE
- NUTS/NUT BUTTER
- SUNSALTED SEEDS
- PROTEIN SHAKE WITH COCONUT MILK
- GRANOLA/POWER BALLS
- AVOCADO/WHOLE FRUIT/ VEGGIES

Beware of bad oils

Portions

complex carbs   protein   healthy fat   snack

PHASE FOUR

WEEK SEVEN GROCERIES

This list includes items you will use for dinner and potentially lunches the next day. Be sure to add in fresh items to make breakfasts and prepare snacks. Organic or local fresh farm raised items are preferred.

Double check your stock pantry list to make sure you have the essentials. If you have made your meat rub, taco seasoning and breading, the "aisle" ingredients will be minimal. Spices can be purchased in larger quantities online.

MEATS

Unless otherwise specified, the recommended serving size will depend on the number of portions. The recommended amount of meat/fish per serving is 1/2 pound.

- [ ] whole chicken or 4 chicken breasts
  (for white chicken chili)
- [ ] 1-2 pounds of grass-fed ground beef
  (for tomato sauce; if you have frozen sauce from week 1, you may omit this ingredient)
- [ ] 2-3 pounds of grass-fed beef (for burgers)
- [ ] white fish or salmon-avoid tilapia
  (for spiced dry rubbed steak)

REFRIGERATED SECTION

- [ ] eggs (1 dozen NEEDED for egg parmesan, purchase additional as needed for breakfast)
- [ ] coconut milk (unsweetened)
- [ ] coconut yogurt (plain/unsweetened; no more than 1-2 grams of sugar)
- [ ] Pecorino Romano cheese
  (check local wholesale clubs for value; for egg parmesan)

AISLE

- [ ] coconut and/or olive oil
- [ ] Dijon mustard
- [ ] pickles (avoid artificial dyes)
- [ ] 4 cans of white beans
- [ ] cumin
- [ ] oregano
- [ ] dried Italian spices
- [ ] coconut flour**
- [ ] almond flour**
- [ ] sunflower seeds**
- [ ] lentils (dried, spouted or 2 cans)
- [ ] silvered almonds (for buttery green beans)
- [ ] apple cider vinegar

**Omit these ingredients if breading is already prepped

WEEK SEVEN GROCERIES

PRODUCE

- ☐ 1 butternut squash (pre-cut and frozen available, for vegetable medley)
- ☐ 1 bunch of asparagus (for vegetable medley)
- ☐ 1 red onion (for vegetable medley)
- ☐ 1 red bell pepper (for vegetable medley)
- ☐ 1 zucchini (for vegetable medley)
- ☐ 1 small bag of carrots (fresh, pre-cut or frozen for lentil soup)
- ☐ 6 fresh onions or 3 bags of frozen onions
- ☐ 1 bunch of collard greens (fresh or frozen for white chicken chili)
- ☐ 2 bunches of cilantro (for white chicken chili and burgers)
- ☐ basil (for tomato sauce)
- ☐ parsley
- ☐ garlic (fresh, jarred or frozen)
- ☐ lemon juice (omit if not making marinade for chicken)
- ☐ 1 spaghetti squash (zucchini can be substituted; base for egg parmesan)
- ☐ green beans (fresh or frozen; to substitute for fries with burger)
- ☐ lettuce for salad (spinach, romaine, mixed greens, arugula, etc.)
- ☐ 1 cucumber (for cucumber and tomato salad)
- ☐ 1 package of grape tomatoes (for cucumber and tomato salad)
- ☐ 2-3 eggplants (for eggplant parm or eggs if you repeat egg parmesan)

This list includes items you will need for dinners and most lunches. Be sure to add items you will need for breakfasts and other members of your household.

DAILY PRIORITIES

Have you ever stopped to consider what you actually do in a day? Planning our daily activities makes us more likely to succeed in accomplishing them. Use this planner to prioritize your upcoming week.

	MONDAY	TUESDAY	WEDNESDAY	THURSDAY	FRIDAY	SATURDAY	SUNDAY
5:00							
6:00							
7:00							
8:00							
9:00							
10:00							
11:00							
12:00							
1:00							
2:00							
3:00							
4:00							
5:00							
6:00							
7:00							
8:00							
9:00							
10:00							
11:00							

SNEAKY INGREDIENTS

HIDDEN NAMES OF SUGAR

- Barley malt
- Beet sugar
- Brown sugar
- Buttered syrup
- Cane juice crystals
- Cane sugar
- Caramel
- Corn syrup
- Corn syrup solids
- Confectioner's sugar
- Carob syrup
- Castor sugar
- Date sugar
- Demerara sugar
- Dextran
- Dextrose
- Diastatic malt
- Diatase
- Ethyl maltol
- Fructose
- Fruit juice
- Fruit juice concentrate
- Galactose
- Glucose
- Glucose solids
- Golden sugar
- Golden syrup
- Grape sugar
- High-fructose corn syrup
- Honey
- Icing sugar
- Invert sugar
- Lactose
- Maltodextrin
- Maltose
- Malt syrup
- Maple syrup
- Molasses
- Muscovado sugar
- Panocha
- Raw sugar
- Refiner's syrup
- Rice syrup
- Sorbitol
- Sorghum syrup
- Sucrose
- Sugar
- Treacle
- Turbinado sugar
- Yellow sugar

HIDDEN NAMES OF MSG

- Ajinomoto
- Anything hydrolyzed
- Any hydrolyzed protein
- Autolyzed Yeast
- Calcium Caseinate
- Calcium Glutamate (E 623)
- Gelatin
- Glutamic Acid (E 620)2
- Glutamate (E 620)
- Natrium Glutamate
- Monosodium Glutamate (E 621)
- Monopotassium Glutamate (E 622)
- Monoammonium Glutamate (E 624)
- Magnesium Glutamate (E 625)
- Sodium Caseinate
- Soy Protein Isolate
- Textured Protein
- Yeast Food
- Yeast Extract
- Yeast Nutrient
- Whey Protein Isolate
- Vetsin

INGREDIENTS THAT OFTEN CONTAIN MSG

- Anything containing enzymes
- Anything enzyme modified
- Any flavors or flavoring
- Anything protein fortified
- Anything ultra-pasteurized
- Barley malt
- Bouillon and broth
- Carrageenan (E 407)
- Citric acid, Citrate (E 330)
- Maltodextrin
- Malt extract
- Pectin (E 440)
- Protease
- Seasoning
- Soy sauce
- Soy sauce extract
- Stock

WEEK EIGHT MEALS

BREAKFAST

These are suggested breakfast items. Breakfast may be substituted with a shake, balanced in proteins, fats and carbs.

EGGS: scrambled, boiled, fried, omelette (add herbs, onions, tomatoes, greens and/or avocado)

FRITTATA MUFFIN

GRAINLESS GRANOLA (1/4-1/3 cup)

GRAINLESS WAFFLES

SHAKE can be used as a meal replacement

CHIA PUDDING (1/4-1/2 cup)

DINNER

You may eat the meals in the order you choose.

PIZZA with salad

PASTA PRIMAVERA, SWEET POTATO NOODLES and salad (rice, spelt, or whole grain noodles in moderation)

CHICKEN FINGERS with **RAW VEGGIES** and Ceasar salad

ROAST BEEF & CAULIFLOWER MASH with salad

BUTTERNUT SQUASH SOUP with salad

PURPOSEFUL LEFTOVERS

DINE OUT to challenge yourself to make great choices.

LUNCH

Lunches should be purposeful leftovers from dinner the night before. Leftovers can be accompanied by :

SOUP

RAW OR COOKED VEGETABLES

BOILED EGG

OLIVES (3-5)

GOAT OR SHEEP MILK CHEESE small amount

FRESH MIXED GREENS topped with protein

SNACKS

These are approved snacks that are optional. Be mindful to combine a protein, a fat and a carbohydrate with snack options.

- CARSON'S CRACKERS
- HARD BOILED EGGS
- SICILIAN SPICED OLIVES
- PECORINO ROMANO CHEESE
- NUTS/NUT BUTTER
- UNSALTED SEEDS
- PROTEIN SHAKE WITH COCONUT MILK
- GRANOLA/POWER BALLS
- AVOCADO/WHOLE FRUIT/ VEGGIES

Beware of bad oils

Portions

complex carbs

protein

healthy fat

snack

PHASE FOUR

WEEK EIGHT GROCERIES

This list includes items you will use for dinner and potentially lunches the next day. Be sure to add in fresh items to make breakfasts and prepare snacks. Organic or local fresh farm raised items are preferred.

Double check your stock pantry list to make sure you have the essentials. If you have made your meat rub, taco seasoning and breading, the "aisle" ingredients will be minimal. Spices can be purchased in larger quantities online.

MEATS

Unless otherwise specified, the recommended serving size will depend on the number of portions. The recommended amount of meat/fish per serving is 1/2 pound.

- [ ] 3 pounds chicken breasts/tenders
- [ ] 3-4 pounds beef roast
- [ ] pizza topping of your choice (read ingredients)

REFRIGERATED SECTION

- [ ] eggs
- [ ] Pecorino Romano cheese
- [ ] 3-4 ounces fresh mozarella (per pizza)
- [ ] sour cream/whipping cream (optional)
- [ ] coconut yogurt

AISLE

- [ ] coconut and/or olive oil
- [ ] pesto sauce with olive oil (for pizza crust)
- [ ] dried Italian spices
- [ ] garlic powder*
- [ ] flax seed*
- [ ] sesame seed*
- [ ] hemp seeds*
- [ ] paprika*
- [ ] coconut sugar*
- [ ] Himalayan salt
- [ ] 1 cup coconut flour**
- [ ] 1 cup almond flour**
- [ ] sunflower seeds**
- [ ] red wine
- [ ] beef broth
- [ ] 1-2 jars of tomato puree
- [ ] rice, spelt or whole grain noodles (option)

*Omit these ingredients if dry rub is already prepped

**Omit these ingredients if breading is already prepped

WEEK EIGHT GROCERIES

PRODUCE

- [ ] 2 butternut squash (pre-cut for soup)
- [ ] 3-4 apples (for soup)
- [ ] 1 small bag of carrots (frozen, ore-cut for soup)
- [ ] 2 heads of cauliflower (1 for mash, 1 for pasta primavera)
- [ ] 2-3 bags frozen cauliflower (for pizza crust)
- [ ] 1 bunch of asparagus (for pasta primavera)
- [ ] 2-3 red bell peppers (for pasta primavera and pizza topping)
- [ ] vegetable noodles (zucchini, sweet potato, butternut squash etc.) (for pasta primavera)
- [ ] 1 purple onion (for pasta primavera)
- [ ] 4 white onions (for roast)
- [ ] 1-2 bags of frozen onions (for soup)
- [ ] 8 ounces of sliced mushrooms (optional, for pizza)
- [ ] 2-3 cups fresh spinach (for pizza topping)
- [ ] fresh basil
- [ ] fresh parsley
- [ ] 2-3 heads of garlic (fresh, frozen, or jarred)
- [ ] lettuce for salad (Romaine, Kale, etc.)
- [ ] sweet potatoes (to cut into noodles)

This list includes items you will need for dinners and most lunches. Be sure to add items you will need for breakfasts and other members of your household.

WEEKS 9, 10 & BEYOND

It was only a short time ago that you were revamping your kitchen. If you are here, you should be proud of you sticking to things! From this point on you will have food freedom! You of course, are welcome to use some or all of the new recipes you have learned. You may also use the knowledge you have gained to substitute unhealthy ingredients for better ones in recipes you have loved for years.

Take this time to work on balancing your macronutrients and feeding your body enough to sustain you through daily activities and exercise but not enough to store excess fat. Try new recipes and be creative enjoy the changes you have made. Remember when you get off track the best time to get back on the road to success is in your next meal. Forgive yourself, don't be too hard on yourself. You don't have to wait until next week, next month or next year to get healthy, just your next meal!

When experiencing the Keyes Ingredients' nutritional protocol, weight loss is a common side effect. This is due to limiting processed and refined foods and replacing them with whole, nutrient-dense foods. Though most people lose a little weight on the program, there are a few inhibitors to losing weight. Our bodies are self-healing, self-regulating masterpieces and will do what they need to do to protect themselves.

Listed below are a few of the reasons why people might hit a plateau in weight loss, or find it difficult to lose weight altogether.

DEFICIENCY:

Nutritional deficiency is common with the processed and refined ingredients that have made their way into our food sources. Refined foods lack essential vitamins and minerals, therefore, there is a need for quality supplementation.

PHASE FIVE

WEEKS 9, 10 & BEYOND

TOXICITY

Toxins come from the environment, chemicals in our food and in the many products we use on our skin. The bottom line is -- toxins that enter our bodies live in our fat cells. Detoxification is essential to rebooting our metabolism and losing weight. A couple of ways to get rid of toxins are to enjoy organic whole foods and to educate ourselves on the environmental toxicities, and then avoid them as much as we can.

PROPER REST

Rest does a body good. Sleep is very important, and good quality uninterrupted sleep is essential for proper metabolism and weight loss. Seven to eight hours of quality sleep each night is best.

CHRONIC STRESS

Stress is extremely common. We have all experienced it and it is never fun. Knowing what triggers our stress and preventing those triggers is very wise. It is not easy, and it takes time. Learning methods for planning and preparing not only our meal times and our meals, but also our day-to-day lives, will help us to avoid complete chaos and live in a more orderly fashion. Cortisol is the stress hormone. Chronic cortisol release is unhealthy and often responsible for the stubborn "belly fat" we all find unsightly.

Continue to make better choices to maintain your better quality of life. A healthy lifestyle just doesn't happen it follows the law of cause and effect. And healthy lifestyle includes proper nutrition, consistent exercise, eliminating toxicity, correcting deficiencies, a good nights sleep and a balanced nervous system. Chiropractic focuses on spinal restrictions and misalignments that may potentially be creating under stress thereby impeding your body's ability to express full health. Go forth making great choices and being an example of how to live life with vitality.

SUSTAINABLE SUBSTITUTE LIST

Changing the focus from what we **CAN'T EAT** to **ALL THE THINGS WE CAN**

IODIZED SALT

Pink Himalayan Salt

REFINED SUGAR
Coconut Sugar
Raw Honey
Organic Maple Syrup
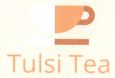

VEGETABLE OIL
Olive Oil
Coconut Oil
Grass Fed Butter
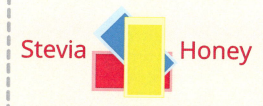

ALL PURPOSE FLOUR
Coconut Flour   Almond Flour
Arrow Root Flour

COFFEE
Dandy blend herbal beverage

Tulsi Tea

ARTIFICIAL SWEETENER
Stevia   Honey

SODA, FRUIT JUICE
Kombucha
Sparkling Water
Coconut Water
Fresh Citrus Sparkling Water with Balsamic/Apple Cider Vinegar
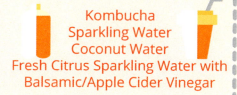

ALCOHOL
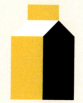
Kombucha

COW'S MILK DAIRY
Sheep/Goat Milk Dairy
Coconut Milk/Yogurt

BREAD OR PIZZA
Sprouted Grain Bread

Cauliflower Crust
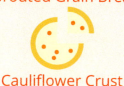

POTATOES
Rutabaga
Squash
Cauliflower
(Mashed)
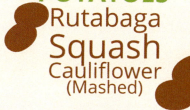

"REGULAR" PASTA
Vegetable Pasta   Shirataki Noodles

Ancient Grain Noodles
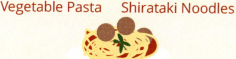

CRACKERS
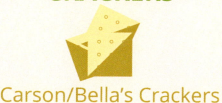
Carson/Bella's Crackers

CHIPS
Nuts   Carson/Bella's Crackers
Seeds

CEREAL
Grainless Granola
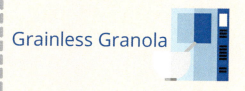

BREADCRUMBS
Ground Sunflower Seeds
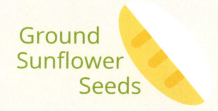

COCOA
Cacao
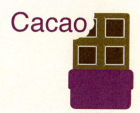

ARTIFICIAL FLAVORS
Fresh Herbs
Dried Spices
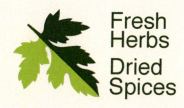

ULTIMATE KITCHEN LIST

VEGETABLES
- Artichokes
- Arugula
- Asparagus
- Bell Peppers
- Broccoli
- Broccolini
- Brussels Sprouts
- Cabbage
- Carrots
- Collard Greens
- Cucumbers
- Eggplant
- Garlic
- Green Beans
- Kale
- Shirataki Noodles
- Mushrooms
- Onions
- Peppers (all kinds)
- Pumpkin
- Potatoes
- Radishes
- Romaine Lettuce
- Spinach
- Squashes
- Sweet Potatoes
- Swiss Chard
- Turnip Greens

FATS/OILS
- Butter (pastured)
- Coconut Oil/Milk
- Ghee
- Olive Oil
- Palm Oil
- Nut Butters
- **NO CANOLA OIL**

WILD CAUGHT FISH
- Anchovies
- Bass
- Cod
- Grouper
- Haddock
- Halibut
- Herring
- Mackerel
- Mahi Mahi
- Red Snapper
- Salmon
- Sardines
- Seabass
- Trout
- Tuna
- **AVOID TILAPIA**
- **AVOID SHELLFISH**

MEAT
- Beef
- Bison
- Chicken
- Duck
- Eggs
- Lamb
- Turkey
- Quail/ Wild Game
- Venison/ Wild Game
- **AVOID PORK**
- *(organic/grassfed)*
- Powdered Collagen
- Protein powder (quality)

FRUITS
PREFERRED
- Avocados
- Blackberries
- Blueberries
- Grapefruits
- Lemons
- Limes
- Raspberries
- Strawberries
- Tomatoes

IN MODERATION
- Apples
- Apricots
- Bananas
- Cantaloupe
- Cherries
- Mangos
- Nectarines
- Oranges
- Papayas
- Peaches
- Pears
- Plums

LIMITED
- Grapes
- Pineapples
- Watermelon

GRAINS
- Brown/Wild Rice
- Kamut
- Quinoa
- Rolled Oats
- Rice Pasta
- Spelt
- Steel cut oats

ULTIMATE KITCHEN LIST

DAIRY
- Coconut Cream
- Coconut Milk
- Coconut Yogurt
- Cows Milk (Raw)
- Cows Cheese (Raw)
- Goats Milk
- Goats Cheese
- Kefir
- Pecorino Romano
- Raw Cream

(limited, raw, or low temperature processed is best)

CONDIMENTS
- Apple Cider Vnegar
- Balsamic Vinegar
- Baba Ganouj
- Coconut Aminos
- Cacao
- Vanilla Extract
- Almond Extract
- Guacamole
- Hummus
- Lemon Juice
- Lime Juice
- Mustard
- Pink Himalayan Salt
- Salsa
- Tamari

BEANS
- Black Beans
- Chickpeas
- Kidney Beans
- Lentils
- Navy Beans
- Pinto Beans
- White Beans

SPICES/HERBS
- Basil
- Black Pepper
- Cayenne Pepper
- Chili Pepper
- Cilantro
- Cinnamon
- Cloves
- Cumin
- Dill
- Fennel
- Garlic
- Ginger
- Mint
- Mustard Seeds
- Nutmeg
- Oregano
- Paprika
- Parsley
- Rosemary
- Sage
- Tarragon
- Thyme
- Tumeric

NUTS & SEEDS
- Almonds
- Cashews
- Chia (Black/White)
- Flax
- Hemp
- Macadamia
- Pecans
- Pistachios
- Pumpkin
- Sesame (Black/White)
- Sunflower
- Walnuts

SWEETS
- Coconut Sugar
- Coconut Nectar
- Maple Syrup
- Raw Honey
- Dark Chocolate

BEVERAGES
- Almond Milk
- Cashew Milk
- Coconut Kefir
- Coconut Milk
- Coconut Water
- Cultured Whey
- Herbal Teas
- Kombucha
- Raw Vegetable Juices
- Sparkling Water
- Spring Water

A Comprehensive Weekly
MEAL PLANNER

	Monday	Tuesday	Wednesday	Thursday	Friday	Saturday	Sunday
Breakfast							
Lunch							
Dinner							

DAILY JOURNAL

Good Morning!

I am thankful for...

Flush Those Toxins!

Breakfast & Supplements

Time:

☐ Supplements

1 hour after breakfast I felt ☐ fatigued ☐ energized ☐ other

Snacks

Lunch

Time:

☐ Supplements

1 hour after lunch I felt ☐ fatigued ☐ energized ☐ other

Snacks

Dinner & Supplements

Time:

☐ Supplements

1 hour after dinner I felt ☐ fatigued ☐ energized ☐ other

Exercise

☐ Cardio ☐ Posture

☐ Strength ☐ Mobility

☐ Walk ☐ Other

Bedtime

Wind Down ☐

Relax/Meditate ☐

No Screens ☒

LET'S TALK ABOUT YOU!

1. Is your Job…
    a. Sedentary *A walk or stretch every 45-60 minutes is beneficial and helps circulation & posture*
    b. Active
    c. Combination of both

2. Do you wake up tired?
    a. Always *Proper sleep affects weight loss (7-8 uninterupted hours is recommended)*
    b. Sometime
    c. Never

3. Do you eat breakfast?
    a. Daily
    b. Often
    c. Sometimes *Ask when they eat if they skip*
    d. Never *Ask when they eat if they skip*

4. How many meals a day do you eat?
    a. 2 Large
    b. 3 Moderate
    c. 5 Small

5. You have fixed mealtimes?
    a. Yes
    b. No *Fixed meal times help maintain blood sugar and insulin levels*
    c. Mostly

6. How often do you eat processed (boxed) foods?
    a. Several time a day *inflammatory, added sugars, empty calories, cravings*
    b. Several time a week *inflammatory, added sugars, empty calories, cravings*
    c. Once in a while
    d. Never

7. How many servings of fruit do you have in a day? _____ *Fruit has natural sugar, 15 grams is recommended to maintain a healthy weight*

8. How many servings of vegetables do you have in a day? _____

9. Do you eat dairy products? *Dairy will be removed & reintroduced during your journey*

Yes   No

10. When consuming Dairy is it organic or raw?

Organic   Raw *Organic or Raw is best, otherwise dairy free.*

LET'S TALK ABOUT YOU!

11. Do you eat meat?

Yes   No *Make sure you are getting good quality protein*

12. When you consume meats/eggs are they farm raised or organic?

Yes   No *Advise on GMO's and antibiotics*

13. How many meals a week do you eat out? _____ *Refined sugar and salt in restaurant foods. Choose wisely, but try to eat at home.*

14. Do you snack in between meals? *You may require snacks due to uncontrolled blood sugar. Goal is to have meals sustain until next meal.*

Yes   No

15. Typical snacks are: *Fruit and nuts are a better choice*
    a. Fruit
    b. Vegetable
    c. Nuts
    d. Seeds
    e. Processed foods (boxed)
    f. Junk food (candy/chocolate)
    g. Juice
    h. Others

16. How many hours a week do you exercise? _____
Exercise is essential. 4-6 hours per week is a great goal. Variety is key.

17. When eating a meal, I am…
    a. Sitting with others
    b. Sitting alone
    c. Standing *Brain does not register eating*
    d. On the go
    e. In front of T.V., computer or other media device *People will eat 2x as much*

18. My consumption includes (check all that apply)
    a. Water
    b. Soda *highly inflammatory & full of empty calories*
    c. Diet soda *neurotoxic*
    d. Tea
    e. Coffee *limit 1-2*
    f. Juice *unless fresh, limit*
    g. Energy drinks *Have unhealthy stimulants*

19. How many Alcoholic drinks do you consume in a week? _____
    2 drinks 2 times a week is suggested

LET'S TALK ABOUT YOU!

20. Do you use artificial sweetener? *If yes, must substitute immediately*

   Yes   No

21. Do you ingest GMO's? (Genetically Modified Foods) *We will learn about GMO's and why to avoid in week 7*

   Yes   No   Not Sure

22. Do you like to cook? *Are you willing to try recipes with limited ingredients?*

   Yes   No   Indfferent

23. How many in your household to cook for? _____
Use this question to help portion recipe

24. Do you suffer from (circle all that apply) *Possible gluten or grain intolerance mostly caused from processed foods*
    a. Gas
    b. Bloating
    c. Indigestion
    d. Digestive upset
    e. Skin rashes

25. Do you use tobacco in any form? *If yes stop immediately. Warn of increased risk of cancer and heart disease*

   Yes   No

26. How many hours' sleep does you average? _____   Is it interrupted? Y / N
Poor sleep does not allow cell regeneration or weight loss

27. How do you cope with/manage stress?

_____

28. Do you feel you are aware of the amount of calories and or macronutrient in food?

   Yes   No *You will be by the end of our journey. A calorie is not a calorie. Quality counts.*

29. Are you familiar with chiropractic care?

   Yes   No

Your nervous system is being freed up from inner stressors in combination with the proper nutrition and toxin elimination. Chiropractic adjustments free your nervous system from inner stresses. Interference of nervous system signals result in a lot of different symptoms and not always pain.

REFERENCES

FOR MORE INFORMATION...

Optimal Health:
The Makers Diet by: Jordan Rubin
Nutritional and Physical Degeneration by: Weston Price
The Metabolic Typing Diet By William Wolcott and Trish Fahey
Anti Cancer by: David Servan-Schriber MD, PHD
Grain Brain by: David Perlmutter, MD
Brain Maker by: David Perlmutter, MD
Always Hungry by: David Ludwig MD, PHD
The Whole Soy Story by: Kaalya T. Daniel PHD, CCN
The Dorito Effect by : Mark Schatzker
The Omnivore's Dilemma Michael Pollen
In Defense of Food Michael Pollen
Eat Fat Get Thin by: Mark Hyman

Raising Healthy Kids:
Healing The New Child Epidemics by: Kenneth Bock MD
Little Sugar Addicts by: DesMaisons Eating Your Child
What's Eating Your Child by: Dorfman

World renound Wellness Experts I trust:
Dr. Joe Mercola, D.O.
Dr. Josh Axe, D.C.
Dr. Mark Hyman, M.D.

All of these well researched doctors have websites, social media and blogs you can learn a lot from.

Content by Michelle Keyes
Clinical content advisory by Dr. Kevin Keyes, D.C.
Photography by Vince Mims
Book designed by Camilo Monroy
Edited by Ashley Smith
Designed in Adobe Illustrator
Typefaces used: Avenir Next & Brim Narrow

WEEK 1 QUICK TIPS

PLAN YOUR SHOPPING DAY, PREP DAY & PENCIL IN THE MEAL PLANNER

1. Lemon-chicken topped Ceasar salad
2. "Spaghetti" with meatballs & salad (made with spaghetti squash, miracle noodles or zucchini noodles)
3. Chicken soup & salad
4. Sesame crusted salmon & vegetable medley (chicken or other fish may be substituted)
5. Beef stew & green salad
6. Purposeful leftovers
7. Dine out or at a friend's to challenge yourself to make great choices

Choose your meals, check your grocery list and cross off what you do not need to purchase based on meal selections. Shop & chop, prep your meals!

COOKING TASKS:

- ☐ Make the tomato sauce
- ☐ Make lemon chicken marinade & refrigerate
- ☐ Make the chicken soup
- ☐ Cut & prep your vegetable medley
- ☐ Make beef stew (takes five hours to cook)
- ☐ Make Ceasar dressing

TIPS:

- ☐ Brown beef while sauce simmers
- ☐ Chicken can be marinated for 2-3 days
- ☐ Cut vegetables for soup, refrigerate
- ☐ Cut vegetables for medley, refrigerate
- ☐ Cut vegetables for stew, refrigerate
- ☐ Will keep 10-12 days

QUICK TIPS

Chopping soup ingredients the night before is a time saver. You can also purchase pre-chopped, fresh or frozen ingredients. Thaw meats beforehand if necessary. Consult your meal plan and recipes for what to take out. Empty your dish washer and sink. Have dish cloths, aprons, towels and paper towels handy. You may want to pull out all pots, pans and utensils you plan on using. Wash your hands, roll up your sleeves start the music and start cooking!

Arrange your ingredients on your counter in groups of what is needed for each meal.
You may have several ingredients that overlap. If they are out and easily accessible it will make it more efficient. Prep a garbage can close by and a counter top garbage bowl on your counter.

On the day you serve the meals:

Lemon-chicken topped Caesar salad:
Grill the already marinated chicken, toss the lettuce in dressing, sprinkle with Pecorino Romano and fresh pepper, top with chicken. Remember to omit croutons

"Spaghetti" with Meatballs & Salad: (made with spaghetti squash, miracle noodles, or zucchini noodles)
Bake your spaghetti squash and shred it or sprialize your Zucchini noodles.
Heat your sauce and meatballs.

Chicken Soup & Salad: Warm the soup through, DO NOT boil. Prep your salad.

Salmon & Vegetable Medley: (chicken or other fish may be substituted) Thaw the salmon, season and bake
as per recipe. Roast already prepared vegetable medley. Prep salad (option: use additional caesar dressing to do a side Caesar)
Beef Stew & Green salad: Warm the stew and top with fresh dill. Prepare your salad.

Salmon & Vegetable Medley: (chicken or other fish may be substituted) Thaw the salmon, season and bake
as per recipe. Roast already prepared vegetable medley. Prep salad (option: use additional caesar dressing to do a side Caesar)

Beef Stew & Green salad: Warm the stew and top with fresh dill. Prepare your salad.

WEEK 2 QUICK TIPS

PLAN YOUR SHOPPING DAY, PREP DAY & PENCIL IN THE MEAL PLANNER

1. Taco salad (beef or chicken) with a cilantro lime dressing or creamy cilantro dressing
2. Minestrone & Salad (feel free to add chicken or beef to the minestrone)
3. Dry-rub Chicken with carrots, onions and a Garden salad
4. Almond-crusted white fish, Vegetable medley, sautéed spinach and Tomato caprese/avocado
5. Grass Fed rib-eyes with vegetable of your choice and cauliflower mash
6. Purposeful leftovers
7. Dine out or at a friends to challenge yourself to make great choices

Choose your meals, check your grocery list and cross off what you do not need to purchase based on meal selections. Shop and chop. Prep your meals.

COOKING TASKS:

- [ ] Make the cilantro lime dressing
- [ ] Season and cook taco meat
- [ ] Make Minestrone
- [ ] Make tomato reduction minestrone
- [ ] Oil & dry rub the chicken
- [ ] Make the "breading" for fish/chicken
- [ ] Dry rub the steaks

TIPS:

- [ ] Can be stored in fridge all week
- [ ] Store in sealed container in fridge
- [ ] Prepare protein (optional)
- [ ] Chop carrots, celery and onions
- [ ] Quarter carrots and onions
- [ ] Mix ahead (portion and freeze extra)
- [ ] Extra rub will keep well in the pantry

QUICK TIPS

Chopping soup ingredients the night before is a time saver. You can also purchase pre chopped fresh or frozen ingredients. Thaw meats before hand if necessary. Consult your meal plan and recipes for what to take out. Empty your dish washer and your sink. Have dish cloths, aprons, towels and paper towels handy. You may want to pullout all pots, pans, and utensils you plan on using. Wash your hands, roll up your sleeves start the music and lets cook!

Arrange your ingredients on your counter in groups of what is needed for each meal. You may have several ingredients that overlap, If they are out and easily accessible it will make it more efficient. Prep a garbage can close by and a counter top garbage bowl on your counter.

On the day you serve the meals:

Taco salad: Warm the taco seasoned meat or sautée your chicken. Assemble the salad. Top the lettuce, tomato, cucumber and green onion salad with the warm meat. Garnish with avocado, pico de gallo and your cilantro lime dressing. Use a grated hard boiled egg to substitute the cheese and a few pumpkin seeds for a crunch.

Minestrone & Salad: Heat the soup through and add optional protein. Serve with a salad.

Dry-Rub Chicken with carrots, onions and a Garden salad: Combine rubbed chicken, carrots and onions (we OMIT potatoes this week) in a roasting pan. Roast at 450 for 1 hour. Remove lid to bronze up. There is a crockpot option on the recipe.*Be sure to make a chicken broth with the carcass of the chicken you will need it in week 3 for lentil soup.

Almond-crusted white fish, vegetable medley, sautéed spinach and Tomato Caprese: (Pecorino Romano or avocado is substituted for the mozzarella) Dip the fish or chicken in egg, then bread, bake or fry. Roast the vegetable medley, sautée the spinach and assemble Tomato Caprese (or other salad)

Grass Fed rib-eyes with grilled asparagus, roasted red peppers and cauliflower mash: Grill or pan fry your steak or chicken, prep your vegetable, make the cauliflower mash. Side caesar goes well.

WEEK 3 QUICK TIPS

PLAN YOUR SHOPPING DAY, PREP DAY & PENCIL IN THE MEAL PLANNER

1. Lentil Soup & Salad
2. Beef Burgers, Fries & Salad
3. Grilled Chicken/Fish & Vegetable medley or vegetable of your choice & Salad
4. Egg Parmigiana, Vegetable Pasta & Salad (time to use week 1 leftover sauce)
5. White Bean Chicken Chili & Salad
6. Purposeful leftovers
7. Dine out or at a friends to challenge yourself to make great choices

Choose your meals, check your grocery list and cross off what you do not need to purchase based on meal selections. Shop and chop. Prep your meals.

COOKING TASKS:

- ☐ Make Bolognese or Tomato Sauce
- ☐ Brown Beef for Bolognese Sauce
- ☐ Make Lentil Soup
- ☐ Fry eggs for Egg Parmiagiana
- ☐ Prepare Chicken/Fish
- ☐ Mix and form Beef Patties
- ☐ Cook Chicken for chicken chili

TIPS:

- ☐ Use leftover or frozen sauce
- ☐ Beef can be cooked, frozen and added later
- ☐ Use pre-chopped/frozen veggies
- ☐ Chicken Breast can be used in place of fried eggs
- ☐ Marinade chicken ahead of time
- ☐ 3 lbs of beef makes approximately 12 burgers
- ☐ Chili has the consistency of a soup not a stew

QUICK TIPS

Chopping soup ingredients the night before is a time saver. You can also purchase pre chopped, fresh or frozen ingredients. Thaw meats before hand if necessary. Consult your meal plan and recipes for what to take out. Empty your dish washer and your sink. Have dish cloths, aprons, towels and paper towels handy. You may want to pull out all pots, pans, and utensils you plan on using. Wash your hands, roll up your sleeves start the music and lets cook!

Arrange your ingredients on your counter in groups of what is needed for each meal. You may have several ingredients that overlap, If they are out and easily accessible it will make it more efficient. Prep a garbage can close by and a counter top garbage bowl on your counter.

On the day you serve the meals:

Lentil Soup & Salad: Heat up the soup and prepare a salad.

Beef Burgers & Fries: Grill the beef patties, pull off fresh crisp lettuce for use as a bun, warm up the fries and prepare a small side salad. Toast the buns for those eating their burger with a bun. Use sprouted grain bread as a better option.

Grilled Chicken/Fish & Vegetable medley & Salad: Grill the Protein, roast the Vegetable Mreadedley, and prepare a salad. Tomato Caprese is a great addition and you have all the ingredients.

Egg Parmigiana, Pasta & Salad: Place fried eggs in a pan, add remaining sauce and heat. Prepare the "noodles", top with sauce and prepare a green salad.

White Bean Chicken Chili & Salad: If possible serve this one the night you make it. Heat through and prepare a salad to serve with . Do not add chicken to soup until you plate it if you serve it at a later date.

WEEK 4 QUICK TIPS

PLAN YOUR SHOPPING DAY, PREP DAY & PENCIL IN THE MEAL PLANNER

1. Pasta Primavera & Salad
2. Chicken Fingers & raw veggies served with salad (Caesar is great)
3. Roast Beef, Carrots & Onions with Cauliflower mash
4. Butternut Squash Soup & Salad
5. Cauliflower crust Pizza (a must try) & Salad
6. Purposeful leftovers
7. Dine out or at a friends to challenge yourself to make great choices

Choose your meals, check your grocery list and cross off what you do not need to purchase based on meal selections. Shop and chop. Prep your meals.

COOKING TASKS:

- ☐ Make cauliflower crusts and refrigerate
- ☐ Make Sauce for pizza
- ☐ Prepare and portion pizza toppings
- ☐ Bread the chicken
- ☐ Make the fries
- ☐ Prepare the vegetables for pasta
- ☐ Make the butternut squash soup
- ☐ Dry rub the roast
- ☐ Prepare vegetables for the roast

TIPS:

- ☐ Make individual sizes (1/3 cup) and refrigerate
- ☐ Use leftover or frozen sauce
- ☐ Precook any meat toppings
- ☐ Serve leftovers as Chicken Parmigiana. Add sauce.
- ☐ Leftover fries can be frozen and reheated later.
- ☐ Protein can be added. Chicken is a favorite
- ☐ Use reserved broth from week one.
- ☐ Place in a Ziploc and store in refrigerator.
- ☐ Use Ground Zero dry rub, Roast can cure for five days.

QUICK TIPS

Chopping soup ingredients the night before is a time saver. You can also purchase pre-chopped fresh or frozen ingredients. Thaw meats before hand if necessary. Consult your meal plan and recipes for what to take out. Empty your dish washer and your sink. Have dish cloths, aprons, towels and paper towels handy. You may want to pull out all pots, pans, and utensils you plan on using. Wash your hands, roll up your sleeves start the music and lets cook!

Arrange your ingredients on your counter in groups of what is needed for each meal. You may have several ingredients that overlap, If they are out and easily accessible it will make it more efficient. Prep a garbage can close by and a counter top garbage bowl on your counter.

On the day you serve the meals:

Pasta Primavera & Salad: Roast veggies and prepare protein (optional). Assemble salad.

Chicken Fingers & raw veggies served with salad (Caesar is great): bake or pan fry chicken and prepare salad.

Roast Beef, Carrots & Onions with Cauliflower mash: Sear the roast and let it slow cook all day, prepare the cauliflower mash and a salad.

Butternut Squash Soup & Salad: Warm soup, add topping (optional), prepare a salad.

Cauliflower crust Pizza (a must try) & Salad: Top your crusts with an olive oil pesto, sauce and toppings bake.

THE KEYES MENU

Week 1

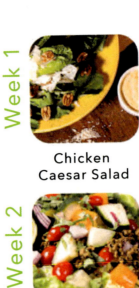

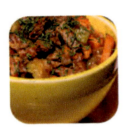 Chicken Caesar Salad

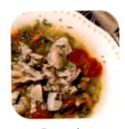 5 Hour Stew

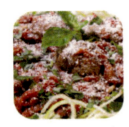 Papa's Chicken Soup

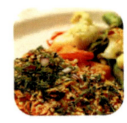 Vegetable Spaghetti & Bolognese Sauce

Sesame Crusted Salmon

Week 2

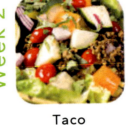 Taco Salad

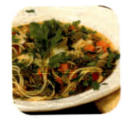 Minestrone Soup

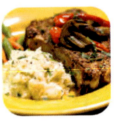 Dry Rub Steak

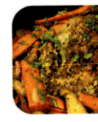 Dry Rub Chicken

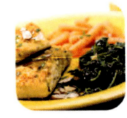 Almond Crusted White Fish

Week 3

 Lentil Soup

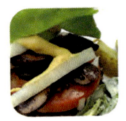 Burgers

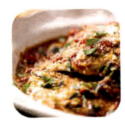 Egg Parmigiana

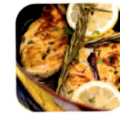 Estelle's Lemon Chicken

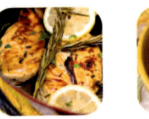 White Chicken Chili

Week 4

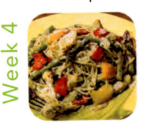 Pasta Primavera

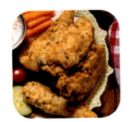 Chicken Fingers

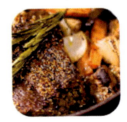 Roast Beef

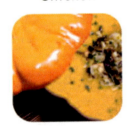 Butternut Squash Soup

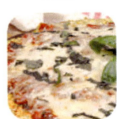 Cauliflower Crusted Pizza

THE KEYES MENU

Week 5

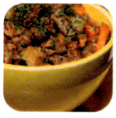 5 Hour Stew

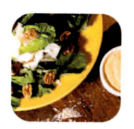 Chicken Caesar Salad

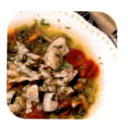 Papa's Chicken Soup

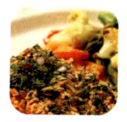 Sesame Crusted Salmon

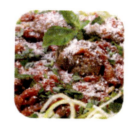 Vegetable Spaghetti & Bolognese Sauce

Week 6

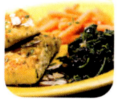 Almond Crusted White Fish

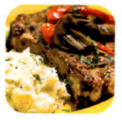 Dry Rub Steak

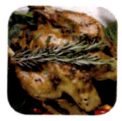 Herb Roasted Chicken

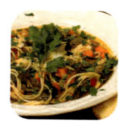 Minestrone Soup

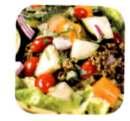 Taco Salad

Week 7

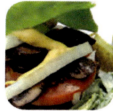 Burgers

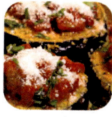 Eggplant Parmigiana

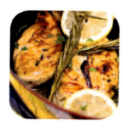 Estelle's Lemon Chicken

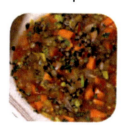 Lentil Soup

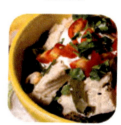 White Chicken Chili

Week 8

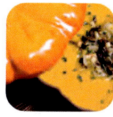 Butternut Squash Soup

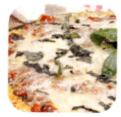 Cauliflower Crusted Pizza

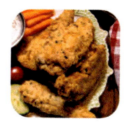 Chicken Fingers

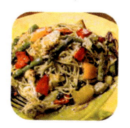 Pasta Primavera

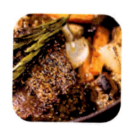 Roast Beef

Made in the USA
Middletown, DE
05 June 2022